AVON

U.S. $6.99
CAN. $9.99

S0-BFE-527

ISBN-13: 978-0-06-077529-2
ISBN-10: 0-06-077529-7

50699

EAN

Foods That COMBAT HEART DISEASE

Includes an Invaluable Anti-Heart Disease Nutrition Counter

The Nutritional Way to a Healthy Heart

LYNN SONBERG

Foreword by JULIUS N. TORELLI, M.D., Consulting Editor

You *can* reduce the risk of heart disease!

Heart disease takes the lives of nearly three thousand Americans *every day!* There are more than sixty-four million sufferers of this dreaded ailment in the United States alone! But there is an easy way to dramatically reduce the risk for men and women alike: eating foods that strengthen your body's defenses so you can *stop heart disease before it starts!*

This invaluable book tells you how.

- Understanding the *new* food pyramid

- Distinguishing between harmful and helpful fats—choosing the *right* fats that actually *protect* the heart

- Replacing refined carbohydrates that wreak havoc on the body's insulin levels with heart-friendly whole grains

- What to look for on food labels

- Charts and tables, recipes and food preparation tips, and an essential nutrition counter to help you win the battle against heart disease

Other Books by the Author

THE COMPLETE NUTRITION COUNTER

THE HEALTH NUTRIENT BIBLE:
THE COMPLETE ENCYCLOPEDIA OF FOOD
AS MEDICINE

THE QUICK AND EASY CHOLESTEROL
AND CALORIE COUNTER

THE QUICK AND EASY FAT GRAM
AND CALORIE COUNTER

THE COMPLETE NUTRITION COUNTER FOR MENOPAUSE

THE FOOD BOOK

Other Books by the Consulting Editor

BEYOND CHOLESTEROL:
THE LATEST SCIENTIFIC DISCOVERIES FOR
PREVENTING HEART DISEASE

Foods That
COMBAT
HEART
DISEASE

The Nutritional Way
to a Healthy Heart

LYNN SONBERG
Foreword by JULIUS N. TORELLI, M.D., Consulting Editor

A Lynn Sonberg Book

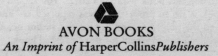

AVON BOOKS
An Imprint of HarperCollinsPublishers

AVON BOOKS
An Imprint of HarperCollins*Publishers*
10 East 53rd Street
New York, New York 10022-5299

Copyright © 2006 by Lynn Sonberg Book Associates
ISBN-13: 978-0-06-077529-2
ISBN-10: 0-06-077529-7
www.avonbooks.com

First Avon Books paperback printing: February 2006

Avon Trademark Reg. U.S. Pat. Off. and in Other Countries, Marca Registrada, Hecho en U.S.A.
HarperCollins ® is a registered trademark of HarperCollins Publishers Inc.

Printed in the U.S.A.

10 9 8 7 6 5 4 3 2

ACKNOWLEDGMENTS

Special thanks are due to Larissa Kostoff, editorial director of Sarahealth Inc., for her invaluable help in researching and writing this book.

CONTENTS

Foods That
COMBAT
HEART
DISEASE

INTRODUCTION

Did you know that if we eliminated all major forms of heart disease we'd live an average of seven years longer?

Seven years.

Heart disease kills. Right now, more than 64 million Americans suffer from it, and each day nearly three thousand Americans will lose their lives to it. That's more than the next five leading causes of death *combined*. Not to mention the fact that, although heart disease was once thought to be primarily a man's disease, heart disease is currently the number-one killer of both men *and* women. Yet the symptoms often differ by sex, as do the causes and the average age of onset. Women, for example, often experience their first major cardiovascular event ten years later in life than men.

What isn't different, however, is what you can change—and that's your diet. Whether you're male or female, the most dramatic prevention of heart disease (and of recurrent heart attack and stroke) starts with your diet. And while many of you may already feel too "full" of information about what and what *not* to eat, in order to maximize heart health you really do need to take stock of the heart-healthy foods available to you. *Foods That Combat Heart Disease* gives you the right information in the right context—information that until now you'd be hard-pressed to find in one easy-to-use, quick reference.

With one in four of us now suffering from it (and 40 percent of us dying from it), it's important to first understand what heart disease is, and what causes it. Also called cardiovascular disease, or CVD, heart disease doesn't just mean heart attack, nor does it refer only to one single disease or condition. Under the umbrella term of cardiovascular disease you'll also find stroke, as well as a whole gamut of health issues, including peripheral vascular disease, or, simply, "blood circulation disease." Peripheral vascular disease occurs when there is an obstruction of blood flow to the limbs (arms, legs, and feet), which creates cramping, pain, or numbness.

It's possible to be born with heart defects leading to some types of CVD, but in most people CVD develops over time. Conditions that affect your heart and blood vessels include the following.

- high blood pressure (this restricts blood flow to the heart)
- high cholesterol (this can lead to atherosclerosis, or hardening of the arteries)

- type 2 diabetes, or insulin resistance (this can increase your risk of heart attack or stroke *fivefold*)

Types of cardiovascular diseases or conditions you might have heard of include the following.

- angina (chest pain caused by deficient blood flow to the heart muscle);
- arteriosclerosis (a hardening of the arteries, also known as "coronary-artery disease")
- atherosclerosis (a narrowing of the arteries due to fatty deposits, known as "plaque")
- congestive heart failure (a weakened heart that's no longer pumping well, which leads to a "backup," and severe fluid retention, called edema)

A landmark international study that involved 262 scientists, 29,000 participants, 52 countries, and a decade of research (published in *The Lancet* in September 2004) reached some striking conclusions; namely, that *90 percent* of the risk factors for heart disease were preventable. The risk factors were ranked according to level of importance, and the complete list is as follows: 1) a bad cholesterol profile, 2) smoking; 3) diabetes, 4) high blood pressure, 5) abdominal obesity, 6) stress, 7) inadequate fruit and vegetable intake, and 8) lack of exercise.

This study definitively proves that poor diet in particular can lead to high blood pressure, high cholesterol, and type 2 diabetes—all of which greatly increase your chances of dying from a heart attack or stroke. No one is saying it's easy, but everyone agrees that you *can* change your diet. So the good news is that overall risk factors for heart disease are within your control. And the first step in taking control is *changing your diet*.

Of course changing your diet won't eliminate other risk factors for heart disease, such as smoking or not exercising (called a sedentary lifestyle). And it won't eliminate the high stress (leading to high blood pressure) that most of us cope with on a daily basis. But it can arm your body with vital nutrients for a healthier heart *in spite* of other risk factors, helping to offset the damage these other factors may cause.

Now that's good news.

Foods that Combat Heart Disease is designed to help you gain the advantage and take charge of what you can control to *stop heart disease before it starts*. If you're recovering from a heart attack or stroke, or are suffering from one of the many problems associated with CVD, the strategies outlined in this book will also help you avoid recurrent episodes, and improve your health in the long term.

So read on. Whether you're a newly health conscious consumer or a heart disease sufferer, this book will tell you what you need to know—in plain language—and in a remarkably easy-to-use format. You'll learn about the foods that adversely affect your heart, and you'll also find more than 2,000 brand name and basic food alternatives, along with the heart-healthy nutrients found in these foods, based on serving size. In addition, you'll learn how to shop for the best heart-healthy foods, and how to store and prepare them to make the most of their nutrients. With three full days of menus and easy-to-prepare recipes, you'll also learn how to plan your daily diet to maximize heart health.

For life.

Are you ready to fight heart disease with every meal? Turn the page—you'll very quickly learn how!

Julius Torelli, M.D.
Director, Integrative Cardiology Center
High Point, North Carolina

CHAPTER 1

FIGHT HEART DISEASE NOW

The evidence is in. You can dramatically reduce your odds of getting heart disease by watching what you put on your plate. Even people with advanced heart disease can actually eliminate their need for surgery by following a heart-healthy diet.

Dr. Dean Ornish led one of the most famous studies in recent decades that documented how heart disease can be halted or reversed through dietary changes, which restricted fat intake to less than 15 percent. His techniques, which also combined other lifestyle modifications (e.g., exercise and stress reduction) were widely published in medical journals. Time and again the results have been replicated by top scientists.

So there's ironclad scientific evidence (more than fifty years of it, actually) to support the link between diet and heart disease.

Early studies made the mistake of slashing daily fat

intake to *half* of the 30 percent that is currently recommended by the American Heart Association. Because these early studies showed such dramatic cardiac risk reduction, Americans were taught a myth: All fat is bad. And then another myth was born: *All* carbs are good.

Today, we know that there are some fats and some carbs that are good for you, and others that are bad for you. But how did these myths get started? Well, once upon a time researchers noted the relationship between the fatty diets that are common in the West and high rates of coronary heart disease. Slash the fat, they reasonably surmised, and you'll also slash your risk of disease. Which is all well and good—so long as what you plan to avoid is *saturated* fat. And don't replace that saturated fat with simple carbohydrates. When you consider that saturated fat represents 40 percent of all fat consumed in the United States, and when you become aware of the effect saturated fat has on your arteries, you start to see the rationale behind the *fat is bad* mantra.

Yet when you look at the Mediterranean diet, which gets 40 percent of its calories from fat and which has been shown to actually *promote* a healthy heart, you begin a much more complicated and yet (ultimately) satisfying education about fat. Mediterranean cultures have long demonstrated surprisingly low rates of heart disease, *despite* their love of wine and the relatively high percentage of fat that they consume.

Why?

Dr. Walter C. Willett decided to rethink the U.S. Department of Food and Agriculture's (USDA) Food Guide Pyramid, which failed to distinguish between healthful, whole-grain carbs and refined carbs, or help-ful fats and harmful fats. He took what we now know about the Mediterranean diet—which contains large amounts of olive oil (the number one source of heart-healthy monounsaturated fat), fish (a great source of heart-protective omega-3 fatty acids) and wine (which in moderation is good for cholesterol)—and combined it with current research. The results, published in *Scientific American* in 2003, are nothing short of revolutionary. They're also very prescient: the USDA is now updating its food pyramid to reflect current thinking about how diet and disease interact.

The science tells us a number of things:

- Refined carbohydrates like white bread and white rice wreak havoc on the body's insulin levels, which increases heart disease risk.
- Replacing these carbs with *whole grains* (see page 20) reduces this risk.
- On the old food pyramid, meat, fish, and poultry were lumped together. We now know that we need to distinguish between *harmful* and *helpful* fats. Red meat and butter, which are high in saturated fat and which therefore increase heart disease risk, should be used *very sparingly.*
- The *right* fats (see page 11) actually protect the heart, and should be consumed at most meals.

What a difference a diet makes. Follow-up studies, wherein subjects ate in accordance with the new food pyramid, demonstrated a 30 percent decrease in heart disease risk among women and a 40 percent decrease among men. And the best part? Instead of focusing primarily on what *not* to eat, or what to *restrict,* Willet's model encourages us to fill our plates with an abundance of foods that actually help the heart. It is for that reason this chapter is structured around foods that *protect* (such as the right fats, the right carbs, the type of fiber that's particularly heart-healthy, and the very best of your heart-healthy vitamins and minerals) rather than *harm.* Naturally, you'll also learn about foods you should avoid, as well as what your cholesterol profile means, if you're at risk for developing high blood pressure, and so on.

The New Food Pyramid

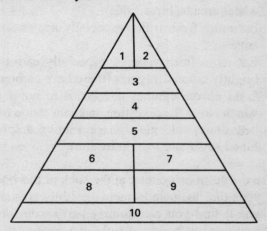

1. Red meat and butter: limit wherever possible.
2. White rice, white bread, potatoes, pasta and sweets: limit wherever possible.

3. Dairy or calcium supplement: 1–2 servings per day.
4. Fish, poultry and eggs: 0–2 servings per day.
5. Nuts and legumes: 1–3 servings per day.
6. Vegetables: in abundance.
7. Fruit: 2–3 servings per day.
8. Whole grain foods: with most meals.
9. Plant oils (particularly olive and other vegetable oils): with most meals.
10. Daily exercise and weight control.

Strategies for Choosing Healthy Carbs

1. Eat lots of plant-based foods.
2. Eat more unrefined whole grains (e.g., whole-wheat breads, brown rice).
3. Eat more fresh fruits, especially apples and oranges.
4. Eat more fresh veggies, especially carrots and brightly colored veggies (these have carotenes).
5. Load up on legumes and beans to boost fiber, which slows the digestion and conversion of carbohydrates into glucose (preventing a spike in blood sugar and then in insulin).

Use the nutrition counter at the back of this book to plan your diet to include more healthy carbs. In no time you'll find you can quickly and easily identify what you need to build the right diet for future heart health.

THE RIGHT FATS

All fats aren't equal. In fact the *right* fats are actually good for you, and have been shown to raise HDL, or "good" cholesterol. We also now know that they're a crucial part of the way our bodies process the phytochemicals they require from various plant-based foods. Moreover, the very valuable nutrients we derive from vegetables are in many cases fat-soluble, so in totally removing the fat from our diets, we're also removing the nutrients, notably vitamins A, D, E, and K.

All fats are known as fatty acids, and in their proper form they nourish our cells. But each molecule of fat contains three different kinds of fatty acids: saturated (solid), monounsaturated (less solid, with the exception of olive and peanut oils), and polyunsaturated (liquid) fatty acids. And it's particularly important, in this case, to distinguish the right from the wrong.

Helpful Fats

Helpful fats promote good health, particularly heart health, so you should be using them often. They include the following.

* *Monounsaturated fats,* which are far and above the most beneficial to your heart. Olive oil best represents this category of helpful fats (along with hempseed oil, it contains the highest amount of them). And olive oil is the reason monounsaturated fats are associated with the Mediterranean diet, which is famous not only for the olive and

the vine (see page 36 for more information) but also for its very low rates of heart disease. Monounsaturated fats protect the heart by lowering levels of bad (or LDL) cholesterol. It's also possible, though as yet unproven, that monounsaturated fats raise levels of good (or HDL) cholesterol. Add to that their proven track record in lowering the risk of insulin resistance and you can see why these are the favorite of our helpful fats. Other examples of foods high in monounsaturated fats include canola, flaxseed, peanut, and avocado oils.

- *Omega-3 fatty acids,* which represent one of the two classes of polyunsaturated fats. Both omega-3 (alpha-linolenic, or ALL, fat) and omega-6 (linoleic, or LA, fat) are polyunsaturated fats, which the body doesn't manufacture on its own and which therefore must be obtained through the diet. But *only one* of these two classes of polyunsaturated fats—omega-3s—is heart-protective. This is largely because omega-6s are so plentiful (too plentiful, in fact) in the western diet. Found in meat, as well as in safflower, sunflower, and corn oils, too much omega-6 fatty acid can actually suppress your immune system and increase your risk of tumors and inflammation.

Not so with heart-protective omega-3s, which are obtained either from plant sources (such as walnuts and walnut oil, flaxseeds and flaxseed oil, soybeans and soybean oil, canola oil, wheat germ, and spinach) or fish (the coldwater variety, such as salmon, mackerel, and albacore tuna).

It's estimated that as many as 99 percent of Americans don't consume enough omega-3s, even though we're getting more than our share of omega-6s. But it's crucial that we find a balance. This is particularly true where the prevention of heart disease is concerned, since omega-3s help to: a) increase our good (or HDL) cholesterol, thereby reducing our risk of heart disease; and b) control hypertension (due to the beneficial effects they have on the elasticity of our artery walls).

The Top 5 Sources of "Helpful" Fat
1. olive oil
2. other plant-based oils such as canola and flaxseed oil
3. seeds
4. nuts
5. coldwater fish (e.g., mackerel, salmon, albacore tuna, sardines)

What You Can Do Now
Look for sources of monounsaturated fats: olive and other vegetable oils (such as canola, flaxseed, peanut and avocado oils), seeds, nuts, and all plant-based foods (with the exception of coconuts). Remember that olive oil in particular is tremendously heart-protective. Also, try to eat more of the following coldwater fish: mackerel, albacore tuna, salmon, and sardines. And don't forget that the key here is balance: tailor your daily fat intake as outlined on the following page.

BALANCING FATS IN YOUR DIET

Type of Fat	How Much to Eat
Total fat	No more than 30% of daily energy requirements
Saturated/polyunsaturated fat	No more than 10% of daily energy requirements
Trans-fatty acids	Limit as much as possible, and keep what you do eat under 3% (which you should factor into the 10% saturated/polyunsaturated fat limit)
Monounsaturated fat	As much as possible (within daily limit)
Plant- and fish-derived omega-3s	A serving, or 1 gm, of each per day (eating 2–4 servings of fish per week will enable you to meet this goal)

HARMFUL FATS

The following are examples of the artery-clogging "harmful" fats you're going to want to avoid. Eating them in excess will increase your risk of cardiovascular problems (or your risk of recurrence, if you've already experienced a major cardiovascular event).

Saturated Fats

Think of them as fats that are solid at room temperature. Not so different, actually, from how they'll look in your arteries, as these fats stimulate cholesterol production in the body. Eating too much saturated fat will make you more susceptible to blood clotting, which increases your risk of stroke and heart attack. Foods high in saturated fat include full-fat dairy products, both processed and fatty meat, lard, butter, margarine, solid vegetable shortening, chocolate, and tropical oils (coconut oil is more than 90 percent saturated).

What You Can Do Now

Saturated fats should be avoided wherever possible, and otherwise consumed only in very small amounts. Nutritionists recommend that saturated fats *plus* trans fats make up no more than 10 percent of a healthy person's daily caloric intake. If you suffer from heart disease, high cholesterol, or diabetes, the recommendation is slightly different—7 percent for saturated and trans fats combined.

Trans Fats

The sneakiest of the harmful-fat family, trans fats are factory-made fats that act just like saturated fat in your body. Bubbling hydrogen gas through vegetable oil creates trans fats, and this process makes the liquid oil (think corn oil) more solid (think margarine). It also prolongs the shelf life of fats, such as polyunsaturated fats, which can oxidize when exposed to air. Not to mention the fact that partly hydrogenated liquid oils, which are basically a pourable shortening, are less greasy tasting. So restaurants, from your best to your most basic, love them, which you probably already know.

There has been a great deal of press lately about the significant quantities of trans fats in our fast foods. Research tells us that just one gram of trans daily (which is ten times *less* than what the majority of us consume on any given day—the equivalent of one chicken nugget or two slices of pizza) will actually increase our risk of heart disease by as much as 20 percent. And studies out of the department of nutrition at Harvard have recently linked trans fats to as many as 33,000 deaths in North America each year.

Exactly why are trans fats so harmful? Well, researchers tell us that trans fats

- increase levels of bad (or LDL) cholesterol.
- decrease levels of good (or HDL) cholesterol.
- increase levels of triglycerides, which are a type of fat produced by the liver and are also obtained in the diet (high levels of triglycerides will put you at greater risk for blood clots).
- increase levels of a substance called C-reactive protein, which in excess can cause inflammation of the blood vessels.

What You Can Do Now

Read your labels. The word you're looking for is "hydrogenated" but you're going to need to be careful, because advertisers routinely claim that such products contain "no saturated fat" or are "healthier" than products high in saturated fat. Or, they're sold with the promise that they've been made with "polyunsaturated" or "monounsaturated" vegetable oil. Either way, if these products contain hydrogenated oils, they might as well be full of saturated fats, because your body really won't know the difference.

According to the U.S. Food and Drug Administration (FDA), we're getting our trans fats from the following sources: 40 percent from baked goods, 21 percent from animal products (like meat and dairy, which contain them naturally), 17 percent from margarine, 8 percent from fried potatoes, 5 percent from potato chips and other salty type snacks, 4 percent from household shortening, 3 percent from salad dressings, and 1 percent from breakfast cereals and candy.

In July of 2003 the FDA opted to include trans fats on the Nutrition Facts panel of conventional foods and some dietary supplements. However, food manufacturers had until January 1, 2006 to comply with this ruling, so you may have been eating trans fats for years without even knowing it. And until recommended daily intake levels for trans fats are established by the National Academy of Sciences, it's best to *limit* foods known to contain them. Either way, saturated and trans fat *combined* should never be more than 10 percent of a healthy person's daily caloric intake (with trans fats never in excess of 3 percent). And ideally you should avoid trans fats altogether.

A NOTE ON MARGARINE VS. BUTTER

When trans fats were added to our watch lists in the late 1980s, margarine was considered one of the highest sources of trans fats. Since then some margarine manufacturers have been offering "healthier" alternatives. Some of these contain no trans fats, others a reduced amount. The latter (or "lighter") varieties are particularly misleading; more often than not they boast a reduction in total fat per serving and yet *still contain trans fats*. As a general rule, a margarine with 9 to 11 grams of fat contains 1–3 grams of trans-fatty acid per serving. And the "hard" margarines—those that look and feel the most like butter—are especially high in trans fats.

However, a stick of butter is about 53 percent saturated fat. So what you gain when you avoid an hydrogenated margarine you most certainly lose when you consume a full-fat butter. The jury's still out in terms of which is better (or which, you might say, is worse). Many experts these days recommend skipping butter altogether and opting, instead, for a trans-fat-free margarine.

What You Can Do Now

If you're a margarine lover choose a brand with less (or no) hydrogenated oils. And if it's butter you prefer, go light—many brands now offer a reduced fat alternative. Better yet, steer clear of both of these questionable bread spreads, and drizzle your foods with heart-healthy olive oil.

Focus Your Approach to Fat

- Opt for fish two to four times per week, and choose the coldwater variety (such as salmon, mackerel, or albacore tuna), as they're high in heart-protective omega-3s.
- Use olive oil for just about everything; Mediterranean cultures even sprinkle it on bread in place of butter, and over pasta (with a little garlic) in place of fattier cream or tomato sauces.
- Be aware that olive oil also "activates" the healthy

carotenes in vegetables, because carotenes are lipophilic. If you don't consume fat along with them (say, in your salads) or at least two hours after eating them, you won't absorb the nutrients they have to offer. So, when dressing salads, olive oil is actually a far better bet than some of the "nonfat" options available today.

- Combine a little flaxseed oil, which is high in omega-3s, with vinegar in salad dressings, and honey mustard or barbecue sauce in marinades.
- Sprinkle chopped nuts or sesame seeds over salads, or choose soy nuts as a healthy snack.
- In general, stick to low-fat and nonfat food choices. The counter at the back of this book will help you determine which food choices are good ones, and also which foods you'll want to avoid.
- Any time you refrigerate animal fat (as in soups, stews or curry dishes), skim the fat from the top before you reheat and reserve. A gravy skimmer will also help skim fats because the spout pours from the bottom, which helps the oils and fats to coagulate on top.
- Powdered nonfat milk has come back with a bang, largely because it's both high in calcium *and* low in fat. Substitute it for any recipes requiring milk or cream.
- Try fruit for dessert. Or, consider a fruit sorbet topped with low-fat vanilla yogurt.
- Pay attention to how you season any low-fat meals. If you do it well, you won't miss the flavor a more fatty alternative provides.

- Protein that's low in fat comes from vegetable sources, such as various grains and beans. Protein that's high (or higher) in fat comes from animal sources.
- Instead of frying, baking, or roasting your meat, broil, grill, or boil it. (Although if you drain the fat first and then cook in water, baking or roasting is fine.)
- With meat, you'll definitely want to trim any of the fat that you can see (both before cooking and before serving).
- Stay away from breaded toppings. Even with lean meat and vegetables, they only add calories.
- Remove skin from chicken prior to cooking.
- Consider the fat content of all your dairy foods. Just as an example, skim milk is fat-free, whereas 1% milk has a 26 percent fat-from-calories content, and with 2% milk, you're looking at 37 percent. Butter gets 95 percent of its calories from fat, and cheese gets 50 percent, whereas with yogurt the number drops to just 15 percent.

THE RIGHT CARBS

Fat, as we've seen, can hurt the heart. But it isn't the only culprit. *What about carbs?* Your body will store carbohydrates (think starches like rice, pasta, bread, and potatoes) as fat if you eat more of them than it can use. In the end, that might make *you* fat also.

Carbs come in two varieties: simple or refined, and complex. Simple carbohydrates are found in foods containing natural sugars (fruits and fruit juices, vegetables, honey, and milk) as well as anything with table sugar. *Refined* carbs (such as baked goods made from white flour as well as white rice and refined pasta) are particularly bad for us, and help make us fat. The former popularity of Atkins and other low carb approaches to dieting signaled the end of a trend that saw people replacing calories from fat with an equal amount of calories from carbs. Too often, however, they chose the "wrong" carbs. If you load up on simple or refined carbs you risk causing a spike in blood sugar and then a spike in insulin. People who load up on simple or refined carbs can eventually develop hyperglycemia and insulin resistance (wherein the body doesn't make enough insulin or else doesn't use the insulin it does make very efficiently). Insulin also keeps the levels of good (or HDL) and bad (LDL) cholesterol, as well as triglycerides, in check. So too many simple or refined carbs can cause your LDL levels and your triglycerides to rise, and your HDL levels to fall, all of which can lead to heart disease.

Complex carbohydrates are more sophisticated because they're made up of larger molecules, and include foods high in fiber, as well as grains and other starches. However, the right carbohydrates are—along with certain fruits and veggies—*whole-grain carbohydrates.* Whole-grain carbohydrates, such as oats, barley, whole wheat, and bulgur, contain every part of the grain. Refined carbohydrates, on the other hand, have been stripped—often of their healthiest, most nutrient-packed components. Whole grains are essential to health, particularly heart health, so it's important that you learn to tell the difference. Any grain products *not* distinguished by the word "whole" on their labels or at the top of their ingredients lists should be avoided. White rice and white pasta should also be avoided.

10 Ways to Reduce Heart Disease with the Right Carbs

1. Have at least one serving of 11 percent oatmeal or high fiber cereals per day.
2. Replace white breads with whole wheat or buckwheat.
3. Eat apples and oranges for daily fruit servings.
4. Replace whole milk or 2% milk with skim milk.
5. Replace white potatoes with sweet potatoes or yams.
6. Replace white rice with brown rice.
7. Have one serving a day of the following beans: lima, butter, green, kidney, soy.
8. Try one of these a week: black-eyed peas or lentils.
9. Use whole-wheat pastas instead of white pastas.
10. Eliminate or reduce sugar from your diet where you can; use sugar substitutes or cut sugar quantities in half.

When you eat the right carbs in the right quantities they convert to glucose, or blood glucose—your body's "fuel." It's only if you eat too much of them (more, for example, than your body can use) that they get stored as fat.

What You Can Do Now

Take a look at what you're eating on any given day, and then compare that with what the nutritionists recommend: 50 to 55 percent carbohydrates, 15 to 20 percent protein, and (as we've already discussed) no more than 30 percent fat. You might also consider the 40/30/30 model. Now known as "The Zone" (because it's said to represent the zone for maximum calorie-burning) this approach to a balanced diet grew out of the research of Dr. Barry Sears. What Sears exposed were the health consequences of diets that were too high in carbohydrates (or, more accurately, too high in *simple carbohydrates*). His solution became the model for The Zone: a diet that derives 40 percent of its calories from carbohydrates, with the remaining 60 percent evenly split between protein and fat.

The Glycemic Index

The glycemic index is designed to help you choose the right carbs. Foods with a high glycemic value (sugary or starchy foods) will convert into glucose faster than foods with a low glycemic value. It follows that foods with a low value convert into glucose slower, which keeps your blood sugar levels more stable and even throughout the day, and keeps you feeling less hungry. You also produce less insulin.

The faster a food converts into glucose, the *higher and faster* your blood sugar will rise, which, as you know, isn't good. This is what causes "sugar crashes" as well as an increase in insulin production, which in turn triggers your appetite. People who eat more foods that have high glycemic values are more at risk for insulin resistance and diabetes as well as heart disease. Conversely, the slower a food converts into glucose, the slower your blood sugar will rise, which, as you know, is better for your health. The glycemic index is also an important tool for people with diabetes, as it helps them choose the right carbs for their meal plans.

This glycemic index, developed at the University of Toronto, Canada, measures the rate at which various foods convert to glucose, which is assigned a value of 100. Foods with higher numbers indicate a much faster absorption of glucose. Use this list as a *sample* only, and remember that it's not an index of food energy values or calories; some low GI foods are high in fat, while some high GI foods are low in fat. Keep in mind, too, that the value assigned to the food will change depending on what else you're eating with it as well as how it's been prepared.

A SAMPLE GLYCEMIC INDEX

Type of Carb	GI Value
Sugars	
Glucose	100
Honey	87
Table sugar	59
Fructose	20
Snacks	
Mars bar	68

Type of Carb	GI Value
Potato chips	51
Sponge cake	46
Fish sticks	38
Tomato soup	38
Sausages	28
Peanuts	13
Cereals	
Cornflakes	80
Shredded wheat	67
Muesli	66
All Bran	51
Oatmeal	49
Breads	
Whole wheat	72
Buckwheat	51
Fruits	
Raisins	64
Banana	62
Orange juice	46
Orange	40
Apple	39
Dairy Products	
Ice cream	36
Yogurt	36
Milk	34
Skim milk	32

Type of Carb	GI Value
Root Vegetables	
Parsnips	97
Carrots	92
Instant mashed potatoes	80
New boiled potato	70
Beets	64
Yam	51
Sweet potato	48
Pasta and Rice	
White rice	72
Brown rice	66
Spaghetti (white)	50
Spaghetti (whole wheat)	42
Legumes	
Frozen peas	51
Baked beans	40
Chickpeas	36
Lima beans	36
Butter beans	36
Black-eyed peas	33
Green beans	31
Kidney beans	29
Lentils	29
Dried soybeans	15

SOLUBLE VS. INSOLUBLE FIBER

Now that you're maximizing the *right* fats and minimizing the *wrong* fats and carbohydrates, would you like to make it even easier?

Consider the benefits of fiber.

Fiber is the favorite of our "good" carbs, and it comes in two types: water-soluble fiber (which dissolves in water) and water insoluble fiber (which actually absorbs water instead of dissolving in it). Though they do differ, both are beneficial. And both take a considerable amount of time to digest in your body, which keeps your blood sugar levels in check and keeps *you* feeling less hungry. Check your hunger and you're also likely to check your intake of the "wrong" fats and carbs.

Insoluble fiber is what promotes regularity (always a good thing, and probably what comes to mind when you think of fiber). It's also a crucial component in the prevention of colon cancer.

But it's soluble fiber that's important to heart health. Experts aren't entirely sure why it does what it does, but they do know that soluble fiber lowers the levels of "bad" cholesterol (or LDL) in the body. One theory is that soluble fiber combines with the bile our livers secrete, forming a gel-like "shield" that traps the building blocks of cholesterol, thus lowering levels of LDL. Whatever causes this reduction in "bad" cholesterol, however, is certainly worth taking seriously.

The Top 10 Sources of Soluble Fiber
 1. Oats
 2. Oatbran
 3. Legumes (e.g., dried beans or peas)
 4. Seeds (all kinds)
 5. Carrots
 6. Bananas
 7. Oranges
 8. Soy products
 9. Wheat bran
10. Flax seeds

What You Can Do Now

Try the sources of soluble fiber above. And, since studies show that people with very high cholesterol stand to benefit the most from them, soybeans are an especially good bet. You can very easily increase your soluble fiber by sprinkling a few tablespoons of raw wheat bran on cereals (or by choosing cereals that have already been fortified with extra fiber), or by sprinkling flax seeds over your green salads. Consider substituting bean dips for sour cream dips, and kidney beans for ground beef; or adding beans and other legumes to soups and chilis. Finally, take a look at the following chart to see how your overall fiber intake measures up. Look for fiber among vegetables, fruits, cereals, grains, and nuts and seeds. The key is to populate your diet with more of it than you may be used to getting. Some of the very best fiber, according to food group, is listed on pages 29–31.

THE FIBER CHART

Cereals	Grams of fiber
(based on ½ cup unless otherwise specified)	
Fiber First	15
All Bran with Extra Fiber	15
Fiber One	14
Granola, homemade (1 cup)	13
All Bran	9.7
Raisin Bran (1 cup)	8
Oatmeal (1 cup)	5
Bran Flakes (1 cup)	4.4
Shreddies (⅔ cup)	2.7
Cheerios (1 cup)	2.2
Corn Flakes (1.5 cups)	0.8
Special K (1.5 cup)	0.4
Rice Krispies (1.5 cup)	0.3

Breads	Grams of fiber
(based on 1 slice)	
Rye	2
Pumpernickel	2
12-grain	1.7
100% whole wheat	1.3
Raisin	1
Cracked-wheat	1
White	0

Fruit	Grams of fiber
Avocado (1 Florida)	18
Raspberries, frozen unsweetened (1 cup)	17

Fruit	Grams of fiber
Prunes, stewed (1 cup)	16
Dates, chopped (1 cup)	13
Pears, dried (10 halves)	13
Raspberries, raw (1 cup)	8
Strawberries (1 cup)	4
Blackberries (½ cup)	3.9
Orange (1)	3
Apple (1)	2
Pear (½ medium)	2
Grapefruit (½ cup)	1.1
Kiwi (1)	1

Beans & Legumes	Grams of fiber
(based on ½ cup unless otherwise specified)	
Kidney beans, red, canned	8
Peas, split, boiled	8
Lentils, boiled	8
Beans, black, boiled	7.5
Pinto beans, boiled	7.5
White beans, canned	6.5
Lima beans, boiled	6.5
Refried beans, canned	6.5
Green beans	2

Vegetables	Grams of fiber
(based on ½ cup unless otherwise specified)	
Lettuce, iceberg (1 head)	7.5
Baked potato with skin (1 large)	4
Vegetables, mixed, boiled	4
Acorn squash	3.8

Vegetables	Grams of fiber
Peas, canned	3.5
Corn, creamed, canned	2.7
Brussels sprouts, frozen, boiled	3
Asparagus (¾ cup)	2.3
Corn kernels	2.1
Zucchini	1.4
Carrots, fresh, cooked	1.2
Broccoli	1.1

VITAMINS AND MINERALS FOR THE HEART

When you opt for foods that are packed with the heart-healthy nutrients outlined in this section, you reap the benefits of the health- and heart-protecting phyto-chemicals that occur naturally in all fruits, vegetables, and grains. So, it's important not to skimp on the foods listed in the third column of the following table.

You'll notice that omega-3 fatty acids make a second appearance here. They deserve it. You may also recognize some of these foods from our previous look at how the right fat, the right carbs, and getting adequate amounts of soluble fiber can benefit the heart. That discussion focused on the *macronutrients* (such as protein and certain fats) experts now know promote good health, particularly heart health. What's remarkable is the heart-protecting *phytonutrients* (such as carotenoids and certain vitamins and minerals) also abundant in each fruit, each veggie, and each serving of whole grains (see following list).

TOP HEART HEALTH VITAMINS

Vitamin A/Carotenoids

Carotenoids have "pro-vitamin A activity"—so your body produces vitamin A from them. They include: alpha-carotene, beta-carotene, beta-cryptoxanthin, lutein, lycopene, and zeaxanthin

Benefit to Heart: Helps to lower cholesterol levels and prevent ischemic (due to a blood clot) stroke. High levels of carotenoids have been shown to reduce the rate of ischemic stroke by as much as 40 percent.

Food Sources: Carotenoids give many of our plants (and even some of our animal foods, such as salmon and shrimp) their colorful hue.

Found in liver, fish oils, egg yolks, whole milk, butter, yellow and orange vegetables and fruits (even tomato sauce is full of them!), red bell peppers, winter squash, sweet potatoes, dark leafy greens, apricots, spirulina, and seaweeds.

Serving Suggestion: At least one serving per day; although many health experts recommend getting 6 milligrams per day of beta-carotene in particular. With foods rich in beta-carotene (such as carrots, pumpkins, and other yellow and orange fruits and vegetables), you're automatically getting other carotenoids as well.

Vitamin C

Benefit to Heart: Protects against heart disease. Taking very large amounts of vitamin C was linked with lower rates of coronary artery disease in an eight-year study at Brigham and Women's Hospital in Boston.

Food Sources: Found in citrus fruits, broccoli, green and yellow pepper, strawberries, cherries, peaches, papaya, guava, cantaloupe, cabbage, tomato, potatoes, leafy greens.

Serving Suggestion: At least two servings per day; though the current DRI for vitamin C is 75 milligrams for women and 90 milligrams for men. Just as an example: 1 sweet raw green pepper has 106 milligrams; 1 papaya, 108; 1 cup frozen, unsweetened peaches, 236; and 1 cup raw Acerola cherries, 1,644.

Vitamin E

Benefit to Heart: Vitamin E has been shown to lower cholesterol by preventing the formation of arterial plaque. In a study of 87,000 nurses taking vitamin E, researchers noted a 46 percent drop in the incidence of heart attack.

Food Sources: Found in nuts, seeds, whole grains, fish-liver oils, fresh leafy greens, kale, cabbage, asparagus.

Serving Suggestion: At least two servings per day; the DRI for vitamin E is 22 International Units (IUs) daily. Just as an example: 1 cup of Total Raisin Bran has 45 IUs; 1 tablespoon wheat germ oil, 39; 1 cup of trail mix, 23; and 1 ounce dry roasted sunflower seeds, 12.

Omega-3 fatty acids

Benefit to Heart: Omega-3s have been shown to increase levels of HDL (or "good" cholesterol), and control hypertension, both of which help to reduce heart disease.

Food Sources: Plant sources: walnuts and walnut oil, soybeans and soybean oil, flaxseed and flaxseed oil, wheat germ and wheat germ oil, canola oil, and green, leafy vegetables (such as spinach).

Marine sources: coldwater fish such as salmon, mackerel, albacore tuna, and sardines.

Serving Suggestion: At least one serving each of both plant-derived and marine-derived omega-3 fatty acids per day.

As an example, a serving of plant-derived omega-3s is a little less than a tablespoon of flaxseeds. A serving of marine-derived omega-3s is about a gram of fish.

However, if you eat coldwater fish 2–4 times per week, and use the recommended oils, you're certain to benefit from these helpful fats.

Potassium

Benefit to Heart: Works with sodium to maintain a normal fluid balance and reduce high blood pressure (when we're not getting enough potassium, our bodies retain sodium and fluid, causing blood pressure to rise).

Food Sources: Found in celery, cabbage, peas, parsley, broccoli, peppers, carrots, potato skins, eggplant, whole grains, pears, citrus, seaweeds.

Serving Suggestion: At least one serving per day—or about 800 to 1,500 milligrams for every 1,000 calories of food. Just as an example: 1 papaya has 781 milligrams; 1 9-inch banana, 742; 2 ounces raw sunflower seeds, 392; and 1 tablespoon wheat germ, 550.

A WORD ABOUT GOOD AND BAD CHOLESTEROL

The recent trans fats media blitz is actually one of the byproducts of more than a decade of research into the relationship between trans fatty acids and cholesterol. One study out of Harvard (which followed more than 85,000 women) found that those who went on to develop heart disease consumed *significantly* more trans fats, which, as you know, lower the good (or HDL) cholesterol while increasing the bad (or LDL) cholesterol in our bodies.

Cholesterol is a waxy fat made by the liver. The body actually needs the cholesterol it produces to insulate nerves and also to make cell membranes and hormones. Problem is, we're also now getting a ton of dietary cholesterol through animal products like meat, poultry, fish, and dairy.

If you have high cholesterol you may experience a "hardening" or "narrowing" of your arteries over time. This is because you've got too much cholesterol in your blood, and the buildup (called plaque) will eventually slow the flow of blood to your heart, significantly increasing your risk of heart disease.

What You Can Do Now

Use the tips in this book to help you choose the foods that will lower cholesterol, and eliminate the ones that won't. The American Heart Association (AHA) recommends that you limit your average daily cholesterol intake to less than 300 milligrams, and make that 200 or lower if you already have heart disease. (Just as an example, one large, raw egg has 215 milligrams of cholesterol—and that's entirely because of the yolk!)

How to Reduce "Bad" Cholesterol

- Limit egg yolks, meat, poultry, fish, seafood, and whole-milk dairy products.
- Eat no more than six ounces of lean meat, fish and poultry per day (and while you're doing that, don't forget about high-quality protein substitutes from vegetable sources, such as beans).
- Choose fat-free or low-fat dairy products.
- Increase your intake of foods that have been proven to lower cholesterol, particularly polyunsaturated fats, fish fats, and soluble fiber.
- Increase foods from plants (fruits, vegetables, grains, nuts, and seeds).

Your Cholesterol Levels:
What the AHA Recommends

You'll want to know your cholesterol levels so that you can tailor your food choices accordingly. Total blood cholesterol is the most common measurement of blood cholesterol, checked through a simple blood test and then measured in milligrams per deciliter of blood (mg/dl).

- A *total cholesterol level* of less than 200 mg/dl puts you at a lower risk for heart disease. Anything higher than this increases your risk. However, levels of 240 mg/dl or higher are a real red flag, and basically mean that your risk for heart disease is now doubled.

- The higher your levels of *HDL cholesterol* the better. At less than 40 mg/dl, you're considered at very high risk for heart disease. However, if you're able to get your HDL cholesterol levels up to 60 mg/dl or greater, the result is actually protective.

- Your *LDL cholesterol* goal depends on the health of your heart. If you don't have heart disease, keep the level below 160 mg/dl, then reduce that number further (ideally, to less than 130 mg/dl) the more at risk you feel you are. If you already suffer from heart disease, your LDL goal should be less than 100 mg/dl.

WINE

Believe it or not, alcohol can raise your levels of good cholesterol, or HDL. The link between wine and heart disease is an old one, but for years it's actually had scientists stumped. This is why, in the late 1980s, researchers decided to look for answers to a culture that *really* worships the vine: the French. It was a perfect choice because the French, who eat such rich food, *still* boast lower levels of heart disease. This is what's known as the French Paradox. And this is what some of the researchers found.

- In the late 1980s, the WHO MONICA project (World Health Organization Monitoring of Trends and Determinants in Cardiovascular Disease) reported major differences in rates of heart disease and deaths from heart disease among the countries/cultures it studied. Participants from the Mediterranean cultures scored low (read "well"), and many researchers attributed this to certain properties present in the wine that they drank.

- In the late 1980s, results of the Copenhagen City Heart Study were published. Researchers in this study followed wine drinkers for up to twelve years, and in this case found that moderate wine drinking was associated with a lower risk of stroke.

Still more evidence exists. But it's difficult to promote the attributes of wine, and in particular, red wine, without a word of caution. So, have some wine—but do take a look at the following.

What You Can Do Now

- Enjoy a glass or two; only make sure it's red. The tannins in red wine, which you won't find in white wine or other liquor, appear to help blood flow and declog arteries.
- Keep in mind that a glass of dry red wine adds about 100 calories to your meal.
- Cook with wine only for the flavor it adds to your food; any of the benefits your heart stands to gain from the wine will evaporate when you cook with it—right along with the alcohol!
- If you really do prefer other kinds of alcohol,

drink them in moderation, and be aware that they don't have the beneficial properties that are unique to red wine. In fact certain alcoholic beverages (and beer is a big culprit here) are also loaded with calories. You might consider acquiring a taste for one of the light beers on the market right now, as well as avoiding the sugary sodas and juices that are often our hard liquor "mix."

THE DASH DIET: PREVENTING HYPERTENSION

If you have high blood pressure, or high blood pressure runs in your family, you need to read this section and follow a DASH diet. Would you believe that high blood pressure, also called "hypertension," affects about 50 million of us? That's right: 1 in 4 adult Americans have it—though it's especially common among those of us who are older (even with normal blood pressure at age 55, we have a 90 percent chance of getting it), or those of us who are African-American.

Blood pressure is recorded as two numbers: X over Y. The X is the systolic pressure (as the heart beats), which is measured over the Y, or diastolic pressure (as the heart rests between beats). Physicians used to frown upon blood pressure readings over 140/90. In fact 120/80 was considered normal. Recently, however, the American Heart Association (AHA) created a new classification—what they call *prehypertension*— to describe those in the borderline range. This now includes people with blood pressures between 120 and 139 (systolic) over 80 to 89 (diastolic). Evidence proves that while those with prehypertension are more likely to move into the hypertension range (where medication will be required), they also respond very well to lifestyle changes aimed at lowering blood pressure.

High blood pressure is most often caused by obesity, inactivity, and stress, though if it runs in your family, or you happen to be African-American, you're at greater risk of developing it. Moreover, once you've got it you're often stuck with it. And uncontrolled, it can lead to heart disease and stroke.

Once again, science has proven that diet affects the health of the heart and can lower the incidence of high blood pressure, or (its medical term) hypertension. Enter the DASH diet. DASH stands for "Dietary Approaches to Stop Hypertension," an eating plan known to lower hypertension. *Anyone who has been diagnosed with high blood pressure should be on the DASH diet.* If your blood pressure is over 130/80, this describes you. Once you're up as high as 160/100, you'll likely be prescribed medication, which you can take in addition to starting the DASH eating program. But DASH is appropriate even if you're in the prehypertensive range and would like to hedge your bets against actually developing hypertension.

It used to be that, on looking for clues about what in the diet affects blood pressure, researchers focused on a variety of *single* nutrients—things like calcium or magnesium. Then, the National Heart, Lung, and Blood Institute decided to conduct a couple of studies that looked at how nutrients work together in our food, as well as their combined effect on blood pressure when consumed as part of a diet low in saturated fat, cholesterol, and total fat, and that emphasizes fruits, vegetables, and low-fat dairy foods. Second, the institute studied how this diet (which became the DASH diet) might further affect blood pressure if sodium intake were then reduced.

The results of these studies (called, simply, "DASH" and "DASH-Sodium") were dramatic. People on the DASH diet alone found their blood pressure was down after just two weeks. And those in the "DASH-Sodium" group, particularly those who already had hypertension, experienced even greater reductions. Clearly, this was a winning combination.

The good news? Not only is hypertension *controllable*, it's also *preventable*.

A Word About Sodium

Salt is sodium chloride. Because our bodies require a balance of sodium and water at all times, sodium is actually a necessary component of good health. However, too much sodium, which in a healthy body is regulated by the kidneys, leads to or aggravates high blood pressure, which, in turn, leads to an increased risk of heart attack and stroke.

How to Follow the DASH Diet

- Reduce sodium intake to 1,500 milligrams per day. If you find this too difficult to manage, aim for 2,400 milligrams per day instead, but make sure it's no higher (and do try to reduce this amount over time).

- Lower saturated fat, cholesterol, and total fat.
- Reduce red meat, sweets, and sugar-containing beverages.
- Include whole-grain products, fish, poultry, and nuts.
- Emphasize fruits, vegetables, and low-fat dairy foods.

A Typical DASH Day

The following table, adapted from recommendations developed by the Heart, Lung, and Blood Institute, is based on 2,000 calories per day. You can vary the number of recommended daily servings in any food group depending on your caloric needs. For example, if your caloric intake is higher, increase the number of servings both of foods you want to reduce (such as fatty foods) and foods you want to emphasize (such as fruits and vegetables). However if your caloric intake is lower, *decrease* the number of foods you want to reduce by one or more servings, but keep the foods you want to emphasize (again, such as fruits and vegetables) at similar amounts.

SERVING RECOMMENDATIONS FOR THE DASH DIET

Food Source	Serving Suggestion
Grains and grain products	7 to 8 servings per day, with 1 serving being the equivalent of a slice of bread or a ½ cup cooked rice, pasta, or cereal.
Vegetables	4 to 5 servings per day, with 1 serving being the equivalent of 1 cup raw, leafy vegetables (or ½ cup cooked vegetables), and 6 ounces vegetable juice.

Food Source	Serving Suggestion
Fruits	4 to 5 servings per day, with 1 serving being the equivalent of 6 ounces of fruit juice, ¼ cup dried fruit, or ½ cup fresh, frozen, or canned fruit.
Low-fat or fat-free dairy foods	2 to 3 servings per day, with 1 serving being the equivalent of 8 ounces of milk, 1½ ounces of cheese, or a cup of yogurt.
Meats, poultry, and fish	2 (or less than 2) servings per day, with 1 serving being the equivalent of 3 ounces of cooked meat, poultry, or fish.
Nuts, seeds, and dry beans	4 to 5 servings per week, with one serving being the equivalent of ⅓ cup nuts, 2 tbsp. seeds, and ½ cup cooked dry beans or peas.
Fats and oils	Aim for 2 to 3 servings per day, with 1 serving being the equivalent of 1 tsp. soft margarine, 2 tbsp. light salad dressing, or 1 tsp. vegetable oil
Sweets (should be low in fat)	5 servings per week, with 1 serving being the equivalent of 1 tbsp. sugar, 1 tbsp jelly or jam, and 8 ounces of lemonade.

What You Can Do Now

To get you started on the DASH eating plan:

- Take it slow. You can gradually increase your consumption of low-fat and fat-free dairy products to three servings a day, for example, by drinking milk with lunch and dinner (instead of, say, soda or beer).
- You can have a serving of vegetables at lunch as well as at dinner; and if you don't eat fruit with those meals, consider trying it as a dessert.

- Try to go meatless at least twice a week. In general, you can up your vegetable intake by choosing recipes (such as stir-frying and some pasta and casserole dishes) that don't focus quite so heartily on meat.
- Limit the meat that you do eat to 6 ounces per day (that's 2 servings), and keep in mind that half of that (3 ounces) is about the size of a deck of cards.
- Maximize your sources of energy and fiber by choosing whole grains wherever possible.

10 Ways to Reduce Sodium

1. Use the counter to track the sodium content in all your foods.
2. Keep in mind that sodium occurs naturally in foods only in very small amounts.
3. Wherever possible, use reduced-sodium or no-salt added products. These days, even cereal manufacturers often offer a reduced-sodium alternative.
4. With vegetables, go fresh as often as you can. Otherwise, look for canned or frozen vegetables that don't contain salt.
5. Rinse canned foods, such as tuna, to get rid of excess salt.
6. Don't use salt when you cook rice, pasta, and hot cereals like oatmeal. Also, avoid the instant or flavored varieties, as these usually have added salt.
7. Look for other ways of adding "zest" to your food. Natural flavor enhancers like lemon and garlic are tasty, *healthy* alternatives to salt.

8. Opt for fresh poultry, fish, and lean meat rather than their canned, smoked, processed, or cured (as in bacon or ham) alternatives.

9. On those days when convenience is a must, check the labels of "ready-made" pizzas, canned soups, salad dressings, and so on. Most contain a lot of sodium but, again, there *are* alternatives.

10. Recognize the "language" of sodium: pickled or cured; soy sauce or broth.

CHAPTER 2

FROM MARKET TO MEALS

Now it's time to leverage what you know about a heart-healthy diet. Understanding which foods help to protect the heart is key. But you're also going to want to know how to select the very best of these foods—the freshest, the tastiest, and certainly the most nutrient-packed—as well as how to store and prepare them. This chapter will help you develop an eye for good produce, meat, and grains. You'll also learn how to interpret the nutrition labels on your packaged food so that the choices you make from this point forward are informed as well as healthy.

The information in this chapter can be used in tandem with the counter at the back of this book. Moreover, the many guidelines geared towards food storage and food preparation are designed as a complement to that counter—allowing you to get the very most out of the informed and healthy choices you're now equipped to make.

FATS AND OILS

As we discussed in Chapter 1, maximizing the *right* and minimizing the *wrong* fats are among the very best ways you can protect the health of your heart. But do remember that a heart-healthy diet is *still* a low-fat diet, because it restricts your calories from fat to 30 percent of your daily caloric intake. And while *what* you consume is key to trimming the fat from your foods, how you prepare those foods (the types of heart-protective oils you choose to use, for example), is also crucial to low-fat eating. To minimize fat, especially harmful fat, consider the following at the grocer's and in the kitchen.

- Olive oil is always a good choice because it's 74 percent monounsaturated, which means it can actually lower cholesterol levels and protect against heart disease. You can use olive oil for just about everything; Mediterranean cultures even sprinkle it on bread in place of butter, and over pasta (with a little garlic) in place of fattier cream or tomato sauces. Olive oil also "activates" the healthy carotenes in vegetables, because carotenes are lipophilic. If you don't consume fat along with them (say, in your salads) or at least two hours after eating them, then you won't absorb the nutrients they have to offer. So, when dressing salads, olive oil is actually a far better bet than some of the "nonfat" options available today.
- It used to be that olive oils were considered too strong for baking. These days, however, there are

many light olive oils on the market that boast a very neutral taste. So there's rarely, if ever, any need to stray from this "protective" cooking tool.

- Other monounsaturated oils are canola, flaxseed, peanut, soybean, and avocado. When cooking for the heart, canola is second in line to olive oil, and is 50 percent monounsaturated.

- Canola oil is extracted from rapeseed, which comes from the cabbage family of plants. There has been some controversy, lately, over its use, as some canola oils are extracted with chemical solvents or high-speed presses to generate heat—and these methods may alter the oil's fatty acid chemistry in ways we have yet to determine. For this reason, you might look for the organic, "expeller-pressed" varieties sold in health food stores.

- Nonstick (and nonfat) cooking sprays are also fabulous for use in low-fat cooking because they completely eliminate the need for butter. These sprays also come in flavors like lemon and garlic, which add a whole lot of taste without the fat. If you coat your saucepan with cooking spray first, you'll only need to add a very small amount of oil for low-fat stir-fries and so on. In most cases, just a teaspoon is enough—especially with the flavored varieties, which pack a wallop of taste.

- For delicious low-fat marinades, fruit juice, garlic, and fresh ginger also add a ton of flavor and moisture without the fat.

- While butter is the ultimate "fatty" dairy product, margarine also has its dangers to the heart, as we saw in Chapter 1. No matter how "unsaturated" the oils are that go into margarine, the process of hydrogenation (which is what turns them into a "spreadable," butterlike product) makes them behave very much like saturated fat in the body. Even experts these days are undecided as to the merits of one over the other. Nutrition expert Dr. Andrew Weil suggests that you think of butter and margarine not in terms of *which is better,* but in terms of *which is worse.* So, the moral of the story? Limit these foods wherever possible and, if you must partake, go for either a butter that is "low-fat" or "reduced-fat" or try a non-hydrogenated/ trans-fat-free margarine (e.g., "Promise" tub). In either case, carefully check the health claims of these products (for more about understanding food labels, see page 60, as well as their ingredient lists and Nutrition Facts panels).

MEATS

Meat is a key player when it comes to fat in the diet. At the grocer's, choose from the following.

- Lean beef (round, sirloin, chuck, loin). Look for "choice" or "select" grades instead of "prime," and lean or extra-lean ground beef (with no more than 15% fat).
- Lean veal, ham, and pork (tenderloin, loin chop) and lean lamb (leg, arm, loin).

- Chicken, Cornish hen, and turkey (all without skins). You can also substitute ground turkey for ground beef in burgers.
- Chicken breast or drumstick instead of chicken wing or thigh.
- Exotic meats, such as emu, buffalo, rabbit, pheasant, and venison. These have less total fat than animals commonly raised for market.
- Fish, fish, and more fish—especially those high in omega-3 fatty acids (mackerel, trout, herring, sardines, albacore tuna, and salmon). Even shellfish, which is higher in cholesterol than most other types of meat, is lower in saturated fat and total fat than most meats and poultry.

When in the Kitchen

- Avoid breaded foods and toppings, which only add calories and refined carbs.
- Trim all visible fat before cooking.
- Remove the skin (as well as the fat under the skin) before cooking. When roasting a whole chicken or turkey, remove the skin just before carving. And definitely don't inject butter or oil underneath the skin before cooking.
- Bake, steam, roast, broil, or stew rather than frying.
- For crispy fish: try rolling in cornmeal before baking.
- For crispy chicken: remove the skin first, then dip in skim milk mixed with some herbs and spices, roll in breadcrumbs, cornflakes, or potato flakes, and bake.

- Skim the fat off pan drippings when making gravy. And for cream sauces, use skim milk and nonhydrogenated soft tub margarine.
- When making dressings or stuffing, add broth or skimmed fat drippings rather than lard or butter, and don't forget to add plenty of herbs and spices for extra flavor.
- Refrigerate meat and meat juices after cooking and *before* adding to stews and soups. That way you can easily trim away any hardened fat.

FRUITS AND VEGGIES

As we discovered in Chapter 1, fruits and vegetables are a crucial component in any diet, and this is especially true if you're gearing your eating towards optimal heart health. In fact, not getting enough of these foods actually *increases* your risk of developing heart disease. The American Heart Association recommends that you get at least five servings per day of vegetables and fruits or fruit juices. Nowadays, many experts put the emphasis on vegetables, urging us to aim for 2–3 servings of fruit per day, and an "abundance" of veggies. Either way, if you prepare and serve these foods correctly, you *only* stand to benefit. Because, while they're packed with heart-healthy vitamins, minerals, and soluble fiber, they're also low in fat and sodium, and they contain absolutely no cholesterol.

You can use the counter to stock your breakfasts, lunches, dinners, snacks, and desserts with the most heart-protective of these foods, but do pay special attention to these.

- Fruits and veggies that are high in soluble fiber. These include legumes, citrus fruit, strawberries, and apple pulp.
- Fruits and veggies that are high in vitamins A (and carotenoids), C, E, and potassium (see Chapter 1 for a complete list of these foods and the heart-healthy nutrients they contain).

And do remember that the trick is to *preserve* the nutrients in fruits and vegetables, which are very sensitive to exposure to light, heat, water, and air.

When Shopping

- Look for the freshest produce available. Once produce starts to brown and wilt (e.g., lettuce) or bruise (e.g., apples, bananas) you can be pretty sure its nutrient value is dwindling.
- To understand how your fruits and vegetables are grown, take the advice of a scientist who was recently quoted in *Gourmet* magazine. Read your labels (or, in this case, your stickers). Apparently those little stickers on your fresh produce list more than just its price. A label with four digits indicates conventionally grown food; a label with five digits starting with an 8 indicates that the food is genetically modified; and a label with five digits starting with a 9 indicates that the food is organically grown.

- If you can't buy fresh, canned fruits and veggies are still a good option (though canning does destroy some vitamin C and B vitamins). However, do check labels for the sodium content of these foods (as well as their frozen or packaged alternatives).
- To evaluate freshness, sniff fruits (such as melons or berries), look for bright colors and, with berries, check the bottom of the box or carton for any evidence of spoiled fruit or staining (which only means that they'll continue to spoil and that nutrient loss has already set in).
- When purchasing leaf lettuce, go for darker shades of green (such as Romaine). Or, if it's a salad mix (such as field greens or mesclun), look for a combination of bright, vibrant greens. This indicates a wealth of carotenoids and other vitamins and nutrients.
- When purchasing vegetables, always opt for variety—in type as well as color. You'll find it's easier to do this if you purchase these foods when they're in season (e.g., root vegetables in the fall) and all their various colors, flavors, and nutrient content are at their peak.
- Try to stay away from packaged, "pre-cut" produce, as cutting only exposes these foods to oxygen, which initiates spoiling and vitamin loss. Moreover, these fancy packets of cut veggies are often far more expensive than regular produce.

Storing and Freezing Your Fruits and Veggies

- When you plan to freeze these foods, refrigerate them immediately (with a few exceptions; namely, bananas).
- Freeze fruits (such as berries and peaches) and vegetables when they're ripe—just after harvest, if possible—because you won't then compromise any of their flavor or nutrition.
- Blanch vegetables (such as asparagus, beans, broccoli, beets, carrots, squash, etc.) just before freezing. This will disarm the enzymes in these foods that work to break down their nutrients. And be aware that steam generally works better than boiling water, as it's gentler on your vegetables' vitamins.
- Eat fresh fruits and vegetables within three to four days of purchasing them, and frozen fruits and vegetables within three to four months of freezing. Nutrient loss occurs either way: after prolonged refrigeration or when the foods have been in your freezer so long that they're exhibiting signs of freezer burn (which compromises both nutrition and flavor).

Preparing Your Fruits and Veggies

- Wash your produce but don't soak it. Soaking causes nutrients to leach out into the water.
- Go raw wherever possible.
- Avoid cutting and dicing, as you'll only expose a larger surface area of these foods to oxygen, which destroys their nutrients.

- Avoid peeling (there's a veritable bounty of nutrients and flavor in those peels!).
- Similarly, cook fruits and vegetables with their skins on.
- Steam or microwave vegetables to avoid adding unnecessary fats. You can also stir-fry (using the heart-healthy oil or cooking spray alternatives discussed later on) or grill them.
- Always cook frozen fruits or vegetables in one step—freezer to saucepan (or microwave). Thawing wakes up all sorts of destructive microorganisms that were frozen right along with your food.
- Use garlic when cooking with vegetables. Garlic has been shown in many studies to lower blood cholesterol levels, thereby reducing risk of heart disease. Dice and cook with olive oil or roast the whole bud (this reduces smell).

THE BULK FOOD BINS

The whole grains and beans that you'll find in the bulk food bins of your grocery or health food stores are less perishable than fruits, vegetables, and baked goods, and usually contain less sodium than the canned or frozen alternatives. These foods are rich in soluble fiber (which means they'll help to lower cholesterol), and high in complex carbohydrates (which means they're packed with vitamins and nutrients). Moreover, they're almost always more affordable than the processed or packaged variety you may be used to eating. And when properly stored, they last forever!

Use the counter to determine which bulk foods are high in soluble fiber, and consider making the following substitutions.

- Dried beans and peas instead of canned or frozen.
- Rolled oat flakes over packaged or "instant" cereal. There are many "stealth" ingredients in things like packaged cereals. For example, Post Select Great Grains (Raisin, Dates, Pecans) Whole Grains Cereals has 1 gram of saturated fat and 0.5 grams of trans fat. Rolled oat flakes, on the other hand, are a great source of soluble fiber and are remarkably easy to make. Just boil and serve as oatmeal.
- Barley. For use in soups (as well as on its own) as a substitute for other starchy fillers. Also high in soluble fiber.
- Brown rice over white. In general, it's always a good idea to opt for those grains that have undergone the least amount of processing. Rice is white because it's been stripped of its husk, germ, and bran layers during processing.
- Whole grains—bulgur, couscous, etc.—as another alternative to your common white starch. Both of these grains, when added to vegetables, can transform a healthy starch into a hearty meal!

A Couple of Reminders
1. Keep stored grains away from moisture of any kind, and always seal them in airtight containers. If you live in a very humid climate, grains will store safely in your fridge for up to one year.

2. Never presoak rice or other grains before cooking them—you'll only wash away their nutrients and, in the process, devitalize the grain. Don't worry about recipes that call for this: presoaking rice, such as basmati and certain other grains, really isn't always necessary and often only leaves the grain (which has absorbed a ton of water) mushy.

BREADS AND BAKED GOODS

Multigrain breads and other baked goods made with whole grains are also good for the heart. Right now dietary fiber among American adults averages out at about 15 grams per day—*half* of the American Heart Association's recommended amount. You already know that certain fruits, vegetables, and legumes are good sources of fiber, especially soluble fiber. But what about bread?

In the case of breads and baked goods the key is to know what you're dealing with. *Read your labels.* One thing you already know for sure is that soluble fiber lowers cholesterol, and it's found in goods baked with oat bran, such as bran muffins and oatmeal cookies, and some multigrain breads. Look for whole-grain breads packed with oats and seeds, such as flax seeds, as these are a source of soluble fiber. But do pay special attention to the ingredients list, as many commercial oat bran products actually contain very little bran. And like other unhealthy baked goods, they may also be packed with sodium as well as saturated and trans fats. As a general rule, the healthy ingredient you're looking for (such as oat bran in this case) should appear high on the list of product ingredients.

Once again, the right carbohydrates are *whole-grain carbohydrates.* Whole grain carbohydrates contain every part of the grain, whereas refined carbohydrates have been stripped—often of their healthiest, most nutrient-packed components. Any baked goods *not* distinguished by the word "whole" on their labels should be avoided. This goes for all your white breads, sugary, cake-type muffins, or white-flour waffles and pancakes *as well as* the host of "wheat" or "multi-grain" products that can't promise they're made with whole grains. Again, *read your labels.* You can tell by the label and ingredients list whether a claim of "whole grain" or "multigrain" is meaningful, or just hype.

Let's take a look at the fiber content of our breads.

Bread	Grams of Fiber*
Prairie Bran	3.5 (contains soluble fiber)
Sunflower Flax	2 (contains soluble fiber)
Oat Bran	1 (contains soluble fiber)
Sesame White	1 (contains soluble fiber)
Whole Wheat Soy	2 (contains soluble fiber)
12-Grain/Multigrain	2.5 (contains soluble fiber)
Rye	2
Pumpernnickel	2
100% Whole Wheat	1.3
Cracked Wheat	1.0
White	0

*Note: refers to insoluble fiber unless otherwise stated.

A Few Reminders

- The "dark" color of a grain doesn't necessarily make it nutritious. Many "enriched" white breads (meaning that the nutrients lost during the processing of the bread have been replaced) have actually been dyed with molasses to get their color.
- As always, read your labels. Many breads are labeled "wheat" but actually contain mostly enriched white flour. Look for 100 percent whole-wheat flour high on the ingredients list. And take calories, trans fats, saturated fats and cholesterol levels into account as well—that way you'll balance your energy intake and avoid less healthy fats.
- Avoid store-bought desserts that call themselves "healthy" just because they're made with unsaturated oils and are low in fat or completely fat free. Most of these are made with refined flour, and are very high in sugar.
- Don't forget to check the trans fat content of the cookies, crackers, and baked goods you *do* eat. A handful of Nabisco Wheat Thins contains 2 grams of trans fats, as much as a Burger King Dutch Apple Pie. There is even a half-gram of this sneaky fat in Quaker Chocolate Chunk Chewy Low-Fat Granola Bars. And two Eggo Buttermilk Waffles have 1.5 grams of trans fats.
- Do check these same manufacturers periodically for newer versions of their "regular" products that are trans free.
- Some manufacturers and restaurant chains are

also enriching their baked goods with soy, which is particularly good for cholesterol levels. Starbucks, for example, now offers "soy-enriched" muffins in most of its stores.

- If you bake, consider quick homemade breads, muffins, pancakes, French toast, or waffles—and try to sneak some soluble fiber into the mix (you can do this with oat bran or by adding certain seeds, such as flax seeds). Use nonhydrogenated margarine (or low-fat butter) and/or oils that are low in saturated fat, fat-free or 1% fat milk, and egg whites or egg substitutes. If you do use egg yolks, do so in moderation, and remember to count them as part of your daily cholesterol.

- When baking homemade bread, choose whole-wheat flour over white, and avoid the self-rising varieties, as they're very high in salt.

- Treat yourself to traditional sweet potato or pumpkin pie. Mix the mashed sweet potato or pumpkin with orange juice concentrate, nutmeg, cinnamon, vanilla, and just one egg—but do avoid the temptation to add any butter to the mixture.

AISLES OF TEMPTATION

For the last ten years or so, it's been a little easier to walk down supermarket aisles—thanks to government legislation requiring the manufacturers of most packaged food to tell us what's inside. Literally. Now, at last, we're not just tempted, we're *informed*. And that makes a world of difference when eating for health—

particularly heart health. The American Heart Association actually participated in the legislation and regulatory process that has made nutrition labeling more useful to consumers. Since 1993, food labels must adhere to guidelines created by the FDA and the U.S. Department of Agriculture's Food Safety and Inspection Service. And since 2003, additional requirements were added to the "Nutrition Facts" panel—ensuring that manufacturers now list "trans fats" or "trans fatty acids" as well. This is great news for consumers, particularly those on a heart-healthy diet. But it's only relevant—not to mention beneficial—if we learn how to interpret those labels.

WHAT'S INSIDE:
UNDERSTANDING THE LABELS ON YOUR FOOD

All labels list "Nutrition Facts" somewhere on the side or back of the package. The "% Daily Values" column offers people perspective on what their overall *daily* dietary requirements should be. It carries a footnote explaining that percentages are based on a 2,000-calorie-per-day diet, and that "a person's individual nutrient goals are based on his or her calorie needs." But it's helpful, because often a nutrient (e.g., sodium) will show up in what appear to be really high numbers (e.g., 100 mg) in a certain food, when in reality 100 mg of sodium is just 4% of the daily value for sodium, which is 2,400 mg.

The % Daily Values column, therefore, explains how high or low a given food is in certain nutrients (such as fat, saturated fat, and cholesterol) by putting it in the context of a whole day's worth of eating. So, in terms of your % Daily Values, what's generally considered *low* is a number of 5 or less (because it represents only 5% of your daily allowance for that nutrient). Consider this a good thing if the label reads <5 for fat, saturated fat or cholesterol, less of a good thing if the label reads <5 for fiber.

On the other hand, "low fat" is a very specific term that means the product contains three grams of fat or less per serving. Likewise, "low calorie" is a specific term that describes a product containing 40 calories or less per serving. (For more on these and other common health claims, see below.)

"Calories" on its own means energy, as in *how much energy* you'll derive from a given food. Calories from fat means, quite literally, *how much energy from fat* a given food contains. These are listed according to serving size, which can be confusing but which is often explained on the label as well (e.g., 1 serving = 1 cup, or 1 serving = 1 bar of a 2-bar granola treat).

Total carbohydrate, dietary fiber, sugars, other carbohydrates (such as starches), cholesterol, sodium, potassium, vitamins and minerals, total fat, saturated fat, and now trans fat are listed in % Daily Values—which is based on the 2,000-calorie-per-day diet that is often recommended by the U.S. government.

The problem is, sometimes this information reads more like code, and it requires that the consumer be able not only to read, but also to have a rudimentary understanding of nutrition, mathematics, a little bit of biology and chemistry and—worst of all—a sense of where and how the product manufacturers might be trying to "sell" their product with misleading health claims.

Light, Lite, and Free:
Understanding Your "Healthier" Alternatives

- *Low fat*: the product contains three grams of fat or less per serving. "Serving" in this case is the operative word, since with some products (like "low-fat" potato chips, where a serving equals six chips), the servings are so small you're likely to eat three times as many of them.

- *Low saturated fat*: the product contains one gram of saturated fat or less per serving (but may still contain significant amounts of trans fat).

- *Low calorie*: the product contains 40 calories or less per serving.

- *Reduced*: the product has 25% less of a given nutrient (e.g., cholesterol) than what you'd find in the standard or "regular" version.

- *Less/ fewer*: the nutrient must be reduced by 25% compared to standard recipes, the "regular" version of a given product.

- *Light*: the product must have half the fat, one-third the calories, or half the salt of the regular product.

- *Free* (as in fat-free, calorie-free or cholesterol-free): the product must have no more than 0.5 grams per serving. The same is true for products listed as "No" (as in no fat) or "Zero" (as in zero cholesterol).

- *Sugar free*: the product must contain less than 0.5 grams of sugars per serving (whereas "reduced sugar" means at least 25% less sugars per serving).

Trans Fats in Our Restaurant Fare

The experts agree: It's almost impossible to avoid trans fats when eating at fast food restaurants because the deep-frying oils used in the restaurant trade are generally hydrogenated. You might even say they're hard to avoid when eating *period,* since we spend, on average, one-third of our food dollars on restaurants and takeout.

But there is hope. First, we can choose to avoid eating deep-fried foods. And second, it's quite possible that labeling for trans fats may soon be mandatory on restaurant menus and at point of purchase in fast-food outlets. McDonald's has reduced levels of trans fats in its European chains, and a group of frustrated consumers has taken legal action in an attempt to bring about a similar change in North America. Already some very forward-thinking restaurants and chains in the U.S. are responding to consumer concern by adopting healthier-choice menus. And manufacturers are stepping up too—trans-free chips from Frito-Lay, such as Cheetos, Tostitos, and Doritos are now available. Does this reflect a growing trend—a move towards healthier, more responsible food production in an industry (particularly in the fast-food industry) that's always been driven by the dollar?

We'll have to wait and see.

In the meantime, take a look at how some of your favorite fast foods add up.

Fast Food	Grams of Trans Fats
Red Lobster's Admiral's Feast (a platter of fried shrimp, scallops, clams, and fish)	22
Large order of Burger King fries	6
A & W onion rings	6
1 Glazed Dunkin' Donut	4
5 small KFC chicken nuggets	4
Burger King Dutch Apple Pie	2
Wendy's 4-Piece Kid's Meal Crispy Chicken Nugget	2.5
2 Generic vegetable spring rolls from Ho Lee Chow Chinese takeout	1.7
Wendy's Big Bacon Classic	1.5
1 Fillet of battered fish from Casey's Fish and Chips restaurant	1.2

CHAPTER 3

THE 10-STEP HEART-HEALTHY DIET

Now that you're armed with an understanding of how to fight heart disease every day with every food you put on your plate, we're going to make things even easier. Enter the 10-Step Heart-Healthy Diet. This is an easy-to-follow daily strategy that pulls together information from the first two chapters of this book, creating a *manageable* dietary model that's based on recommendations from leading health experts and organizations, including the American Heart Association, the National Heart, Lung, and Blood Institute, and The American Diabetes Association.

STEP 1: CUT TOTAL FAT (TO 30% OF DAILY INTAKE) BY EATING HELPFUL FATS

Adjust your total fat intake so that it comprises no more than *30 percent of your daily energy require-*

ments. And while you're at it make sure you don't deny your body the sources of helpful fat that it actually needs. These are your unsaturated fats (monounsaturated and polyunsaturated) and your fish fats (omega-3 oils) and from this point forward they'll be responsible for at least two-thirds of your daily fat intake—or 20 percent of your daily caloric intake. So, if you're currently eating about 2,000 calories on any given day, at least 400 of those calories can come from unsaturated fat (20% of 2,000 is 400). There are nine calories in every gram of fat, which means that what you're now aiming for is about 34 grams of helpful fats. So, by all means, have these fats (olive oil especially, as well as canola, flaxseed, and soybean oils; nuts; seeds; and coldwater fish). And if you're feeling ambitious you can further boost the 20 percent they represent to 25 or even 30 percent of daily intake, thereby totally eliminating harmful fats from your diet.

Are you up for the challenge?

STEP 2: SLASH HARMFUL FATS IN YOUR DIET (TO 10% OR LESS OF DAILY INTAKE)

These are your saturated fats, such as both processed and fatty meat, lard, butter, margarine, solid vegetable shortening, chocolate, and tropical oils. *No more than 10 percent of your daily energy requirements should come from saturated fats*—and even less if you can manage it. Using our 2,000 calorie-per-day dietary model, what this translates into is no more than 10 grams of saturated fat on any given day. To make this goal easier to reach, consider the following.

- Use olive oil or nonfat cooking sprays in the kitchen.
- Substitute fatty or processed meats for leaner meats and fish, and eat no more than 6 oz. of either per day (that's 2 servings, with 4 oz. being about the size of a deck of cards).
- Choose plant-based meat substitutes, such as dried beans, peas, lentils, or tofu (soybean curd) or tempeh (also made with soybeans) in entrees, salads, or soups.

A good rule of thumb: Protein that's low in fat comes from vegetable sources (such as various grains and beans), while protein that's high in fat comes from animal sources.

There is no extra allowance made for trans fats in your 10 percent daily limit of saturated fats. That limit actually represents *all* harmful fats (or saturated and trans-fats combined). So you'll need to be extra wary of the trans fats in your diet. As you already know, this is because trans fats behave like saturated fats in your body. Even worse, there is new evidence to suggest that trans fats are a far bigger culprit in the development of heart disease. Research now tells us that just one gram of trans daily can actually increase our risk of heart disease by as much as 20 percent.

Nutritionists do realize that eliminating trans fats entirely is a very tall order, especially when restaurants and fast-food outlets are not yet required to list them at point of purchase. But *limiting* trans fats is now possible, thanks to new legislation that requires manufacturers to add trans fats to the nutrition labels on their food (to be phased in by January 1, 2006). So, for the first time, consumers will be able to track and compare the trans fat content of their foods using the "Nutrition Facts" panel on the product's package. It's a big step—one the FDA estimates will prevent between 600 and 1,200 cases of heart disease and between 250 and 500 deaths from heart disease each year (starting about three years after the phase-in period for labeling is over). *Read your labels!*

STEP 3: DON'T SKIMP ON DAIRY BUT DO MAKE YOUR 2–3 DAILY SERVINGS LOW IN FAT

Dairy foods are traditionally high in fat. But dairy products are not something you want to eliminate from your diet, as they're a great source of calcium, vitamin D, probiotics, and conjugated lineolic acid (CLA). And there is evidence (although it's as yet unproven) to suggest that people with hypertension are calcium (and potassium) deficient.

A difference of opinion exists these days about just how much dairy we should consume. Dr. Walter C. Willet, author of the New Food Pyramid on page 9, recommends 1–2 servings of dairy or calcium supplements per day. However, participants in the DASH diet studies did very well with 2–3 low-fat dairy foods each day.

Just as an example, let's revisit the number of calories from fat in some of our common dairy foods: Skim milk is fat-free, whereas 1% milk has a 26 percent fat from calories content, and with 2% milk, you're looking at 37 percent. Butter gets 95 percent of its calories from fat, and cheese gets 50 percent, whereas with yogurt the number drops to just 15 percent. So, opting for low-fat (or no-fat) dairy foods can actually make a substantial difference to your total fat intake on any given day.

When the Recipe Calls For ...	Try Using ...
whole milk (1 cup)	1 cup fat-free milk or fat-free milk plus 1 tbsp. olive or canola oil
heavy cream (1 cup)	1 cup evaporated skim milk or ½ cup low fat yogurt and ½ cup plain low-fat cottage cheese
butter (1 tbsp.)	1 tbsp. non-hydrogenated margarine or ¾ tbsp. olive or canola oil
cream cheese	low-fat or nonfat cream cheese is now fairly easily available; a good substitute is 4 tbsp. nonhydrogenated margarine mixed into 1 cup dry low-fat cottage cheese (you may also want to add a tiny amount of fat-free milk)
sour cream	fat-free sour cream is now fairly easily available; low-fat cottage cheese plus low-fat or fat-free yogurt is also a good substitute

STEP 4: ENJOY 2–4 SERVINGS OF FISH EACH WEEK

When baked or grilled, fish is a delicious alternative to meat. Even shellfish, such as shrimp, which are higher

in cholesterol than most types of meat, still contain
less saturated fat and total fat than most meats and
poultry. But you're best choosing from one of the
many coldwater fish for your meals (e.g., canned
mackerel, canned light tuna, salmon, sardines, and herring). These fish are rich in omega-3 fatty acids, which
lower cholesterol and protect against heart disease.
(Other fish, such as swordfish and fresh tuna, are also
high in omega-3 fatty acids, but contain high levels of
mercury.)

Do keep in mind that a typical 3–4 oz. serving of
fish is about the size of the palm of your hand. And,
while increasing your fish intake, reduce your consumption of meat (think smaller servings less often),
and always choose from leaner varieties when you do
partake. Then, consider meat substitutes such as dried
beans, peas, and lentils (to boost fiber) and tofu or tempeh (made from soybeans, which lower cholesterol) in
entrees, salads, or soups.

STEP 5: SELECT THE BEST CONDIMENTS AND OILS

One of the easiest ways to protect your heart through
food is with olive oil. You can use it in virtually all
types of cooking (combining it with a nonfat cooking
spray, if necessary, in the saucepan; or selecting a
"lighter" variety with a more neutral taste for baking),
and in marinades and salad dressings, or drizzled over
whole-wheat pastas and breads. Your next best choices
are the other monounsaturated vegetable oils (such as
canola, soybean, flaxseed, and peanut). Flaxseed oil in

particular, and soybean and canola oils, are heart-smart alternatives. They're rich in omega-3 fatty acids, which have been shown to increase levels of HDL or "good" cholesterol, thereby helping to reduce your risk of heart disease (although certain nuts and seeds, like walnuts, brazil nuts, and sunflower seeds, are also good sources of omega-3s).

On average we get 3 percent of our daily calories from the trans fatty acids in partially hydrogenated vegetable oils. Not only is it possible to eliminate this proven harm to our hearts, it's actually very easy to substitute with foods that help. Heart-protecting olive and other vegetable oils are hands-down your very best alternative.

It's also important to track the sodium content in all your other condiments and oils. Most manufacturers now offer a "light" alternative (which means that it contains half the salt of the regular product) to things like regular soy sauce. And *do* go ahead and season; if you do it well you won't miss the fatty taste of some of the foods you've now chosen to avoid. It's always a good idea to season with plant-based foods such as lemon, garlic, and herbs and spices. They're naturally low in fat and contain only the tiniest amount of sodium—a claim many of the "bottled" varieties aren't likely to match.

STEP 6: HAVE A SERVING A DAY OF POTASSIUM

Potassium (found in raisins, apricots, prunes, citrus, pears, melons, bananas, strawberries, cabbage, spinach, peas, parsley, broccoli, peppers, carrots, potato skins, whole grains, turkey, fish, and beef) helps to maintain the regular, healthy function of the heart and nervous system. There is also evidence to suggest that high blood pressure and potassium (and calcium) deficiency go hand in hand.

Potassium works with sodium to maintain your body's normal fluid balance, keeping blood pressure at acceptable levels. If it's in your cupboard and your freezer and it's packaged, boxed, or canned, there's a good chance it's full of sodium. Even products we'd never consider "salty," such as cereals and cookies, are often quite high in sodium. In fact most of your dietary sodium comes from processed foods—with the remainder added in the kitchen or at the dinner table. And sodium, as you're well aware, can cause blood pressure levels to rise, increasing your risk of heart disease. So, wherever possible, limit your use of salt in the kitchen and at the dinner table, and choose from reduced-sodium or no-salt-added products at the supermarket. As often as you can, go fresh (rather than frozen, canned, smoked, processed, pickled, or cured).

The National Heart, Lung, and Blood Institute recommends limiting sodium intake to no more than 2,400 milligrams each day—the equivalent of about 1 teaspoon of salt. A serving of potassium each day will help you counteract whatever sodium you do consume.

STEP 7: GET MORE FIBER
(BETWEEN 25 AND 30 GRAMS PER DAY)
ESPECIALLY SOLUBLE FIBER

Fiber is obviously an important component of any diet because it slows the digestion and conversion of carbohydrates into glucose (which prevents a spike in blood sugar and then in insulin) and it also helps to promote regular bowel function. But it's soluble fiber that's particularly beneficial to the heart, as it lowers the levels of "bad" cholesterol, or LDL, in the body. Make sure your total fiber content is between 25 and 30 grams per day (most of us hover at around 15 grams). Many foods high in fiber are high in both insoluble and soluble fiber. It's like curds and whey or wheat and chaff. So while the counter definitely counts total fiber, we've gone a step further and have actually indicated which foods are particularly rich sources of *soluble fiber* so you can make better choices. These foods include oats, oat bran, legumes (e.g., dried beans or peas), seeds, carrots, bananas, oranges, soy products, wheat bran, barley, and flaxseeds.

STEP 8: DON'T BE AFRAID OF COMPLEX CARBS

Carbs have been much maligned due to the popularity of Atkins and other low-carb or no-carb approaches to eating. But the right carbohydrates—which, along with your fruits and veggies, are *whole-grain carbohydrates*—are indisputably heart-protective. To combat heart disease nutritionists recommend that you get roughly 40 percent of your daily calories from carbohydrates. Even the more moderate "high-protein" diets, such as the Zone, recommend the 40/30/30 approach.

The key to incorporating carbs into your diet, however, is learning to distinguish complex carbohydrates (such as whole grains, fruits, and vegetables) from simple carbohydrates (such as sugar, honey, or white, starchy stuff like white bread, white rice, and potatoes). When you eat the right carbs in the right quantities you're actually doing your body a favor—providing it with the blood glucose it needs as "fuel." So, enjoy the complex carbohydrates you already know are great sources of fiber, particularly soluble fiber: oat bran, oats, legumes, citrus fruits, strawberries, rice bran, and barley. And *always* opt for whole grains—they lower your risk of coronary heart disease, stroke, diabetes, obesity, diverticulitis, hypertension, certain cancers, and osteoporosis.

But don't forget to watch your intake of simple carbohydrates, as eating too much simple or refined sugar will increase your risk of hyperglycemia (high blood sugar) and insulin resistance, both of which can threaten the heart. The much-quoted Nurses Health Study showed that women who consumed diets with a high glycemic load (full of sugary foods and refined white flour) demonstrated an increased heart disease risk. This comes as no surprise to most nutrition experts. The U.S. Department of Agriculture has been urging the public to reduce consumption of these foods for some time. Problem is, the official food guide pyramid, which was published in 1992, makes no distinction between refined and whole-grain carbohydrates—and actually recommends 6–11 servings per day! What makes Willett's New Food Pyramid (see page 9) so revolutionary is his separation of the two categories of carbs. In the Willett model, white rice, white bread, potatoes, pasta, and sweets appear at the very top of the pyramid and are accompanied by a warning: USE SPARINGLY. Whole-grain foods share the base of the Willet pyramid (along with heart-healthy vegetable oils) and are supposed to be eaten *at most meals*. Again, what a difference a diet makes.

Use the glycemic index in Chapter 1 as well as the counter at the back of the book to help you determine the sugar content of your foods. And, use the vitamins and minerals table in Chapter 1 to help you choose simple carbohydrates that are especially rich in heart-protective nutrients. You should be getting at least five servings of fruits and vegetables a day (with an emphasis on the veggies if you can manage it), and a serving of whole-grain foods at most meals.

STEP 9: EAT MORE SOY PROTEIN (25 GRAMS EACH DAY)

Several years ago, the U.S. Food and Drug Administration (FDA) gave food manufacturers permission to put labels on products that are high in soy protein. The agency had at that point concluded its review of 27 studies that demonstrated the value of soy protein in lowering levels of total cholesterol and LDL (or "bad") cholesterol. Brand new research now ranks a bad cholesterol profile as the number one risk factor *world-*

wide for heart disease—so the benefits of soy are certainly worth taking seriously.

In fact the FDA determined that people who consumed four servings of soy every day were able to lower their level of LDL (or "bad") cholesterol by as much as 10 percent. And, contrary to what you might think, there is no need to eliminate animal-based products such as meat, poultry, and dairy foods from your diet in order to enjoy the benefits of soy protein. However, what is important to remember is that soy comes in many forms. Soybean oil can be found in margarine, mayonnaise, salad dressing, and so on, and it actually *offers no benefit to the heart*. For a soy food to qualify as heart-protective it must contain *soy protein*—at least 6.25 grams of it. And it should also be low in fat, cholesterol, and sodium. Soy protein exists in beneficial levels only in specific foods, such as tofu, soy milk, textured soy protein, tempeh, miso, and soy flour. Foods that contain soybean oil (and there are many of them!) don't qualify as being particularly heart-protective. Here's a closer look at some of the most common forms of soy protein.

- Soy milk, which can be used in place of cow's milk for drinking and in recipes (an 8-ounce glass of plain soymilk contains 10 grams of soy protein).
- Soy flour, which can be used when baking (1 soy protein bar contains 10 grams of soy protein), and because soy flour adds moisture to the mix as well, it also makes a good egg substitute.
- Textured soy protein, which can be used as a meat

substitute (1 soy burger contains 10 to 12 grams of soy protein).

- Tempeh, which is also a good meat substitute (½ cup tempeh contains 19.5 grams of soy protein).
- Miso, which is used for seasoning and in soup stocks (½ cup contains 19 grams of soy protein).
- Tofu, which appears at the end of this list, as it's higher in fat than the other soy food examples. Tofu has a neutral flavor and is available in a variety of textures (4 ounces of firm tofu contains 13 grams of soy protein). Tofu can be stir-fried, mixed into "smoothies," or used as a cheese substitute or even as a cream cheese substitute in dips.

Many grocery stores also now carry soy-enriched baked goods, roasted soy nuts, and soy-based burgers and sausages.

STEP 10: EAT 2–3 SERVINGS OF FRUITS EACH DAY, ALONG WITH AN ABUNDANCE OF VEGETABLES

Until very recently most health experts believed that about half of the risk factors for heart disease were preventable. The startling conclusion of the landmark Canadian-led international study, namely, that *90 percent* of the risk factors for heart disease were preventable, was discussed at length in Chapter 1. But what's interesting in this case is how fruits and vegetables factored into the results of this study. Inadequate fruit and vegetable intake was seventh on a list of eight risk factors. Dr. Willet, in fact, recommends more emphasis on vegetables than fruit. The risk factors were ranked according to level of importance, which demonstrates just how crucial are those five recommended servings. The complete list is as follows: 1) a bad cholesterol profile; 2) smoking; 3) diabetes; 4) high blood pressure; 5) abdominal obesity; 6) stress; 7) *inadequate fruit and vegetable intake*; and 8) lack of exercise.

Not only are fruits and vegetables a great source of fiber and a great alternative on those days you might want to go meatless, they're almost universally low in fat, sodium and cholesterol. And, they're absolutely packed with heart and health-protecting nutrients, such as vitamin A (or carotenoids), vitamin C, vitamin E, and potassium. To benefit your heart, make sure you get at least 2–3 servings of fruits as well as copious amounts of vegetables each day. And to really start reaping the rewards these wonderful foods have to offer, stock your diet with foods from each of the following categories (as well as those you know are high in fiber, especially soluble fiber, calcium, and so on).

1. For vitamin A (carotenoids): leafy greens, yellow and orange vegetables and fruits, red bell peppers, winter squash, sweet potatoes, apricots, spirulina, and seaweeds.
2. For vitamin C: citrus fruits, broccoli, green and yellow peppers, strawberries, cherries, peaches, papaya, cantaloupe, cabbage, tomatoes, potatoes, leafy greens.

3. For vitamin E: leafy greens, kale, cabbage, asparagus.
4. For potassium: celery, cabbage, peas, parsley, broccoli, peppers, carrots, potato skins, eggplant, pears, citrus fruits, seaweeds.

Useful Tips

A single serving of vegetables is about one-half to one cup, cooked. A single serving of fruits is about one half-cup fruit juice or one medium-sized piece of fruit. Airtight containers of fresh fruit (to snack on) and veggies (to add to any entrée or salad) prepared every few days, and then stored in the fridge, will help you meet your goal of at least five servings of these foods each day.

CHAPTER 4

A SAMPLE HEART-HEALTHY MENU

The following three-day menu illustrates what an ideal heart-healthy diet looks like in real life, based on the information provided in Chapters 1–3. This plan is low-fat, yet heart-protective. Tasty and creative, you can see how easy it is to eat hearty! Recipes for items in italics follow this sample menu plan.

Day 1

BREAKFAST
Hearty Seven-Grain Cereal with Raisins
1 slice tofu
1 slice bread, toasted
1 cup soy milk

MID-MORNING SNACK
1 whole orange

LUNCH
Lentil and Barley Soup
Basil and Tomato Salad
1 small carton nonfat yogurt
Baby carrot sticks

MID-AFTERNOON SNACK
Small package of nuts or seeds (e.g., walnuts, almonds, sunflower or pumpkin seeds)
1 banana

DINNER
Asian Salmon Fillet
Brown rice
Spinach and Strawberry Salad with
Basic Balsamic and Olive Oil Dressing
1 glass of dry red wine

Day 2

BREAKFAST
Banana Oat Bran Muffin
Hearty Muesli
½ cantaloupe

MID-MORNING SNACK
1 package dried apricots or raisins

LUNCH
Vegetarian Low-Fat Pea Soup
1 can of Albacore tuna, drained, with lemon wedge and sliced cucumber

MID-AFTERNOON SNACK
  Tomato Blend
  Hummus Dip and whole wheat crackers

DINNER
  Chicken & Green Bean Stir Fry
  Polenta
  1 glass of dry red wine

Day 3

BREAKFAST
  Toasted Raisin Bread
  Fresh Fruit Cup
  Strawberry or Raspberry Tea

MID-MORNING SNACK
  Banana chips

LUNCH
  Feta Fruit Salad
  Ginger Pumpkin Soup
  Baby carrot sticks

MID-AFTERNOON SNACK
  Oh Boy Soy Milkshake

DINNER
  Rotini Turkey Salad
  Lighter Greek Salad
  1 glass of dry red wine

RECITES

(listed in alphabetical order)

ASIAN SALMON FILLET

1 raw salmon fillet per person (about 100 grams)
½ cup chopped onion
½ tsp. olive oil
2 tbsp. light (or low sodium) soy sauce

In nonstick skillet, cook and stir ½ cup chopped onion in ½ tsp. olive oil on medium-high heat for 5 minutes. Top with raw salmon fillet, and drizzle with 2 tbsp. soy sauce. Cover and cook on medium heat for 8 minutes or until salmon is opaque. Each fillet is one serving.

BANANA OAT BRAN MUFFINS

1 cup boiling water
1½ cups All Bran or equivalent
2 cups buttermilk
½ cup canola oil
⅓ cup molasses
2 eggs, beaten
1 tsp. vanilla extract
1 cup whole-wheat flour
1 cup all-purpose flour
1 cup oat bran
½ cup sugar
1 tbsp. baking soda
1 banana, sliced

In mixing bowl, stir boiling water into All Bran; let cool for 10 minutes. Stir in buttermilk, oil, molasses, eggs and vanilla.

In large bowl, combine flours, oat bran, sugar and baking soda. Add buttermilk mixture; add bananas. Stir just until moistened. Place batter in nonstick muffin cups until three-quarters full. Bake at 375 degrees F for 20 minutes or until muffins are firm to the touch. Makes 24 medium muffins.

BASIC BALSAMIC AND OLIVE OIL DRESSING

½ cup balsamic vinegar
⅓ cup water
1 clove garlic, finely minced
1 tsp. granular sweetener or sugar
¼ tsp. salt
pinch freshly ground pepper
¼ cup olive oil
optional: 1 tsp. Dijon mustard
optional: 2 tbsp. finely chopped red onions

Combine all ingredients except oil. Whisk in oil last until well blended. Pour into covered container and refrigerate. Makes 1 cup.

BASIL AND TOMATO SALAD

1 medium tomato, sliced
1 tbsp. dried or fresh basil leaves

Combine ingredients and drizzle with *Basic Balsamic and Olive Oil Dressing*. Makes one serving.

CHICKEN & GREEN BEAN STIR FRY

3 boneless, skinless chicken breast halves (about ¾ lb.)
1 tbsp. light (or low sodium) soy sauce
2 tsp. cornstarch
¼ tsp. freshly ground pepper
2 cups diagonally cut fresh green beans
1½ cups diagonally cut sliced celery
4 green onions, diagonally sliced
1 small sweet red pepper, thinly sliced
2 tsp. canola oil (or no-taste olive oil)
1 tbsp. minced fresh gingerroot
2 cloves garlic, minced
¼ cup salt-reduced chicken broth

Cut chicken into strips. In small bowl, combine soy sauce, cornstarch and pepper; stir in chicken and set aside.

In microwaveable casserole, cover and cook green beans, celery, onions and red pepper with 1 tsp. water on high (100%) for 3 minutes or until vegetables are barely tender.

In wok or large nonstick skillet, heat oil over medium-high heat; stir-fry gingerroot and garlic for 30 seconds. Add chicken and cook for 5 minutes or until all pink has disappeared.

Add vegetable mixture and broth; cook and stir for 3 minutes or until all ingredients are heated. Makes 4 servings or 5 cups.

FETA FRUIT SALAD

1 cup torn red leaf lettuce and watercress
½ medium pear
½ small orange, sliced
1 tbsp. crumbled feta cheese

Combine all ingredients and drizzle with *Basic Balsamic and Olive Oil Dressing*. Makes one serving.

FRESH FRUIT CUP

¼ pink grapefruit, sectioned (orange can be substituted)
4 red seedless grapes
½ kiwi fruit (strawberries can be substituted)
¼ small banana, sliced
¼ cup low-fat yogurt, any flavor
½ cup toasted wheat germ
½ tsp. ground cinnamon

Combine all ingredients and serve. Makes one serving.

GINGER PUMPKIN SOUP

1 can pure pumpkin (19 oz)
3 cups low-salt chicken broth (homemade or canned;
  vegetable broth can be substituted)
½–1 tsp. ground ginger
¼ tsp. salt
¼ tsp. white pepper
1 cup low-fat milk
¾ cup low-fat plain yogurt
¼ cup chopped fresh parsley

In medium saucepan, combine pumpkin, broth, and ginger; and to taste, salt and pepper. Heat slowly for about 15 minutes, stirring occasionally. Stir in milk and heat to serving temperature. To serve, top each bowl with 2 tbsp. yogurt and chopped parsley. Makes 6 servings.

HEARTY MUESLI

2 cups large-flake rolled oats
½ cup oat bran
¼ cup sunflower seeds
¼ cup slivered almonds
¼ cup toasted wheat germ
¼ cup raisins

In medium bowl, combine all ingredients except raisins. Stir well. Spread on baking sheet and bake in 350 degree F oven for 15 minutes. Cool completely. Stir in raisins; store in tightly sealed container. Makes 12 servings of ½ cup each.

HEARTY SEVEN-GRAIN CEREAL WITH RAISINS

1 cup large-flake rolled oats
1 cup 3-grain cereal (commercially sold 3-grain cereal
typically has cracked wheat, cracked rye and whole
flax; found in health food stores)
1 cup whole-wheat flakes
½ cup oat bran
½ cup cream of wheat
½ cup raisins

Combine rolled oats, 3-grain cereal, whole-wheat flakes, oat bran, and cream of wheat. Store in tightly sealed container. Makes 16 servings.

For a single serving: combine in microwaveable bowl ¼ cup dry cereal mix and ¾ cup water. Microwave uncovered on high (100%) for 2 minutes; stir. Microwave on low (30%) for another 3 minutes. Let stand 2 minutes and serve. Sprinkle with raisins.

For stovetop method, combine water and dry ingredients and bring to a boil. Reduce to medium heat and stir for 5 minutes. Cover and remove from heat. Stir and serve. Sprinkle with raisins.

HUMMUS DIP

¼ cup tahini sauce (this is sold in most supermarkets
or health food stores)
⅓ cup lemon juice
2–4 medium garlic cloves
19 oz. can chick peas (garbanzo beans) or 2 cups
cooked chick peas
3 tbsp. chopped fresh parsley or cilantro

Place tahini, lemon juice, and garlic in food processor. Blend until smooth. Drain beans, reserving liquid. Add beans. Blend until mixture is creamy. Add 2–4 tbsp. of bean liquid from can, or lemon juice to thin out mixture. Makes 4 servings.

LENTIL AND BARLEY SOUP

1 tbsp. olive oil
1 large leek (white part only), thinly sliced
1 cup chopped onion
3 cloves garlic, minced
6 cups low-salt beef broth (homemade or canned)
4 medium-sized carrots, cubed
2 stalks celery with leaves, sliced
¾ cup red or green lentils, washed
¾ cup barley, washed
½ cup tomato sauce (canned or homemade)
2 bay leaves
1 tsp. dried rosemary
1 tsp. dried oregano
½ tsp. salt
¼ tsp. freshly ground pepper
sprig of chopped fresh parsley

In large soup pot, heat oil on medium-low heat; cook leek, onion, and garlic, covered, for 10 minutes. Add remaining ingredients, cover and bring to a boil. Reduce heat and simmer 40 minutes or until barley is tender, stirring occasionally. Discard bay leaves. Serve, sprinkled with parsley. Makes 9 cups (or 9 servings).

LIGHTER GREEK SALAD

½ medium tomato, wedged
4 cucumber slices
1 inch cubed feta cheese
2 tsp. lemon juice
½ tsp. olive oil
¼ tsp. dried oregano

Combine all ingredients and serve. Makes one serving.

OH BOY SOY MILKSHAKE

¾ cup soy milk (vanilla or plain)
2 tsp. instant coffee
2 tsp. artificial sweetener
1 tsp. unsweetened cocoa powder
dash vanilla extract
2 ice cubes

Combine all ingredients in a blender until smooth. Makes one serving.

POLENTA

(Note: this fine yellow "cornmeal mush" is packed with B6, niacin, and fiber; a great substitute for potatoes or rice)

½ cup polenta
2¼ cups water
Pinch of salt

In medium saucepan, bring water and salt to boil. Reduce heat to low and slowly whisk in polenta to reduce lumps. Cook slowly for 4 to 5 minutes, whisking constantly or until smooth and thickened, with all liquid absorbed. Serve your main dish on top, as the polenta will soak up the flavors of the main dish. Makes 4 servings.

ROTINI TURKEY SALAD

1½ cups uncooked colored rotini

DRESSING:
2 tbsp. cider vinegar
2 tbsp. light soy sauce
1 tbsp. olive or sesame oil
1 small clove garlic, crushed
1½ tsp. minced ginger root
1 tsp. granulated sugar
pinch of freshly ground pepper

SALAD:
2 cups cubed cooked turkey
1 cup diagonally sliced snow peas
½ medium sweet red pepper, cut into thin strips
½ cup sliced canned water chestnuts
½ cup sliced celery

In large pot, cook pasta according to package directions, until tender but firm. Drain well and cool. Set aside.

Prepare dressing by whisking together dressing ingredients in separate bowl.

Prepare salad by combining all ingredients in separate

bowl. Add pasta and dressing, and toss well. For best results, cover and refrigerate for at least 2 hours for flavors to combine. Serve cold. Makes 6 cups (or about 4 servings).

SPINACH AND STRAWBERRY SALAD

1 package baby spinach, prewashed
1 carton strawberries, sliced

Combine ingredients with *Basic Balsamic and Olive Oil Dressing*.

TOMATO BLEND

2¼ cups tomato juice
¼ low-fat plain yogurt
1½ tsp. Worcestershire sauce
1½ tsp. fresh lemon juice
¼ tsp. freshly ground pepper
(optional) dash hot pepper sauce
3 lemon slices

In blender, combine all ingredients except lemons. Blend until smooth. Pour into ice-filled glass and garnish with lemon slices. Makes 3 servings.

VEGETARIAN LOW-FAT PEA SOUP

1½ cups dry split peas
5 cups water
1–2 bay leaves
1 tsp. salt
1–2 cloves garlic, minced
1 stalk celery, chopped
1 large carrot, sliced
1 leek, sliced
1 tsp. marjoram
1 tsp. basil
1 tsp. cumin

Combine all ingredients in large soup pot, bring to boil and simmer for 3 to 4 hours. Makes 6 servings.

CHAPTER 5

THE HEART-HEALTHY NUTRITION COUNTER

Foods That Combat Heart Disease is the only one-stop guide to the heart-protective substances that already exist in our everyday foods. In it you'll find information about calories, total fat, harmful fats (saturated and trans fats) as well as the right fats (polyunsaturated fats, monounsaturated fats, and omega-3 fatty acids), carotenoids, fiber, sugar, potassium, and sodium. This counter (see pages 107–247) provides nutrient content for basic foods, brand-name foods, health foods, and fast foods, and we hope it will revolutionize the way you select, prepare, and enjoy your foods.

HOW TO FIND YOUR FOODS

If you're trying to locate a given food, look for it alphabetically under its food category. For example, if you're looking for beets, turn to the table of contents, where you'll see an alphabetized listing of food categories, and find "vegetables and legumes." Turn to the page in question (where the vegetable listings begin) and then look under "B" for beets. Specific vegetables are also listed alphabetically, so you'll have no problem locating *beets*. And under *beets,* you'll then be able to choose from a number of options, such as raw, cooked, canned, pickled, etc. These designations make it possible for you to compare the nutrient content of different preparations quickly and easily.

Included in the categories in the counter are *dinners* and *entrees.* Dinners represent entire meals, which usually means that they include an entrée (like fish or chicken), a side dish (often a vegetable), and dessert. Entrees, however, represent *only* the principal food in a meal, such as a pork chop or lasagna.

The counter also includes a fast-food category that's very deliberately set up for easy navigation. Under fast foods, food items are listed alphabetically in sections like breakfast foods, burgers, desserts, Mexican foods, sandwiches, pasta, pizza, poultry, and so on. This makes it possible for you to crosscheck the nutrient quality of, say, a Burger King sandwich with a similar offering from McDonald's.

But fast-food items (and other treats, such as cookies, cakes, and ice cream) are included in the counter as a point of reference only. Obviously you're going to want to limit these foods—and opt instead for nutritious alternatives. To that end, the counter includes "healthier" versions of brand-name products (e.g., low-fat cakes and ice cream) wherever possible. And,

most importantly, the counter teaches you how to identify these healthier alternatives yourself—by isolating
the *helpful* and the *harmful* nutrients in all your fresh
and processed foods.

HOW TO IDENTIFY YOUR
HEART-HEALTHY NUTRIENTS

Each food entry lists the following information in this
order: food name, serving size, caloric content, and the
amount of each of the following (mostly in grams, milligrams or micrograms): total fat, saturated fat, polyunsaturated fat, monounsaturated fat, trans fat, fiber,
sugars, carotenoids, potassium, omega-3 fatty acids,
and sodium. Let's take a closer look.

Serving Size
Serving size refers to the standard amount of food
suggested by the U.S. Department of Agriculture
(USDA) as well as the food industry.

Calories
The "calories" designation represents the amount of
energy that is provided by one serving. This value can
be used to help you accurately plan your meals if
you're trying to lose weight *and* to benefit your heart.
Diets that limit caloric intake to between 1,200 and
1,500 calories per day are generally considered appropriate for long-term weight reduction.

Saturated Fat

Saturated fat is the artery-clogging harmful fat you should aim to avoid, as eating it in excess will increase your risk of cardiovascular problems, or your risk of recurrence if you've already experienced a major cardiovascular event. Saturated fat is fat that is solid at room temperature. Foods high in saturated fat include both processed and fatty meat, lard, butter, margarine, solid vegetable shortening, chocolate, and tropical oils.

No more than 10 percent of your daily energy requirements should come from saturated fats. Given the standard 2,000 calories-per-day dietary model, this translates into a maximum of about 10 grams of saturated fat per day.

Saturated and trans fat *combined* should never be more than 10 percent of a healthy person's daily caloric intake (with trans fats never in excess of 3 percent). And ideally you should avoid trans fats altogether.

Read your labels. The word you're looking for is "hydrogenated" but be aware that advertisers routinely claim that hydrogenated products contain "no saturated fat" or are "healthier" than products high in saturated fat. Or, they're sold with the promise that they've been made with "polyunsaturated" or "monounsaturated" vegetable oil. Either way, if these products contain hydrogenated oils, they might as well be full of saturated fats, because your body won't know the difference.

Polyunsaturated Fat

Together with monounsaturated fat and omega-3 fatty acids, polyunsaturated fat should comprise two-thirds of your daily fat intake. Given the standard 2,000 calories-per-day dietary model, this means that sources of healthful fats (what we call the *right fats* in Chapter 1), should tally in at around 400 calories per day (20% of 2,000 is 400). There are nine calories in every gram of fat, which means that what you're now aiming for is about 34 grams in total of the "right" fat.

There are two classes of polyunsaturated fat: omega-3 (alpha-linoleic, or ALL, fat) and omega-6 (linolenic, or LA, fat). But *only one* of these two classes of polyunsaturated fats is heart-protective—omega-3s. Which is why omega-3s are listed separately in the Heart-Healthy Nutrition Counter. See "Omega-3 Fatty Acids" on page 103 of this chapter for information about how to obtain this helpful fat through diet. And be aware that too much omega-6 fatty acid, found in meat, as well as in safflower, sunflower, and corn oils, can actually suppress your immune system and increase your risk of tumors and inflammation.

Monounsaturated Fat

Together with polyunsaturated fat and omega-3 fatty acids, monounsaturated fat should comprise two-thirds of your daily fat intake. Given the standard 2,000 calories-per-day dietary model, this means that sources of the right fats should tally in at around 400 calories per day (20% of 2,000 is 400). There are nine calories in every gram of fat, which means that what you're now aiming for is about 34 grams in total of "good" fat.

Monounsaturated fat is the very best of the right fats because it can actually help to *lower* cholesterol levels and protect against insulin resistance. Foods high in monounsaturated fats include olive, canola, flaxseed, peanut, and avocado oils.

Trans Fat

Trans fats should be avoided altogether if possible or limited to at most 3 percent of calorie intake. They are formed during hydrogenation, a chemical process that takes relatively healthy unsaturated vegetable oil and turns it into an artery-clogging solid fat. Some of the most popular commercially produced foods in the United States are high in trans fats, including cookies, cakes, breads, crackers, potato chips, french fries, breakfast bars, packaged dinners—and especially fast food. When this book went to press, quantitative data on the trans fat content of foods was not yet available, but as of January 2006, the FDA requires this information to appear on a product's nutrition facts panel. We have used a "+" symbol to indicate a food contains some trans fat and "++" to indicate a product is high in trans fats.

Fiber

Fiber, which is only found in plant foods, is a crucial component in any diet because it aids in digestion and bowel function. And soluble fiber in particular is both health- and heart-protective, helping to lower levels of "bad" cholesterol (or LDL) in the body.

Because soluble fiber is present in fewer foods, the

counter tracks total fiber, and then measures it in grams (gm). Where it lists a foods that contains soluble fiber (such as oats, oat bran, legumes, seeds, carrots, bananas, oranges, soy products, wheat bran, and flax) you'll notice this designation: *SOL. This means that the food is high in soluble fiber, and is therefore important to heart health.

In general, look for foods that pack at least 2.5 to 3 grams of fiber per serving. And make sure your total fiber content is between 25 and 30 grams per day (most of us currently get around 15 grams). To achieve this goal, increase your consumption of fruits and vegetables, and choose foods high in complex carbohydrates (particularly *whole-grain carbohydrates* such as brown rice and pasta and whole-grain breads).

Sugars

Overindulgence in simple sugars (such as products with added sugar or starches that convert quickly into glucose) can lead not only to weight gain, but also to high blood sugar and insulin resistance—both of which increase your risk for heart disease. Sugars in this case are counted in grams so that you can easily see the "total sugars" in your foods. However, you'll notice that this number fluctuates. When the "total sugars" value is unavailable, a value is given for "natural sugars." Any product that contains natural sugars, such as maltose (grains), fructose (fruits and vegetables), lactose (milk products), and so on, may have no added sugar, but still contains natural sugars, and therefore has grams of sugar we can count.

Use the information in the "sugars" category to avoid or limit simple sugars in your diet, and to ensure that you're getting the right carbs in the right quantities. This information can also help you choose the most nutritious brands of your favorite food items (a breakfast cereal, for example, should contain between 0 and 5 grams of total sugars, though you can always add sugar to taste). To combat heart disease nutritionists recommend that you get 40 percent of your daily calories from carbohydrates. It's important to remember, however, that the *right* carbs are *whole-grain* carbs. They lower your risk of coronary heart disease, stroke, diabetes, obesity, diverticulitis, hypertension, certain cancers, and osteoporosis.

Carotenoids

Carotenoids give many of our plant foods (and even some of our animal foods, like salmon and shrimp) their colorful hue. They also help to lower cholesterol levels and prevent ischemic (due to a blood clot) stroke. In fact, high levels of carotenoids in the diet have been shown to reduce the rate of ischemic stroke by as much as 40 percent. And, as an added bonus, every time you load up on foods that are particularly high in carotenoids you're shoring up a powerful defense against cancer, too.

Try to get at least one serving per day; although many health experts recommend getting six milligrams per day of beta-carotene in particular. With foods rich in beta-carotene (such as carrots, pumpkins, and other yellow and orange fruits and vegetables) you're automatically getting other carotenoids as well. However, remember that this is an absolute minimum. Always eat a variety of brightly colored fruits and vegetables. And do follow the recommendations of the new food pyramid, which urges us to consume an *abundance* of veggies and 2 to 3 servings of fruit each day.

The counter designates the amount of carotenoids in foods either by micrograms (mcg) or milligrams (mg), and highlights specific carotenoids as follows: alpha-carotene (AC), beta-carotene (BC), beta cryptoxanthin (BCR), lutein and zeaxanthin (LU+Z), and lycopene (LYC).

Potassium

As you know, potassium helps to maintain the regular, healthy function of the heart and nervous system. And it works with sodium to regulate your body's normal fluid balance, keeping blood pressure at acceptable levels.

Potassium is counted in milligrams herein. However, potassium is present in what are considered *beneficial* levels only in very specific foods. So, choose your foods carefully. And do remember that in this case *more* is definitely *better*—you should aim for at least one serving per day of potassium (or about 800 to 1,500 mg for every 1,000 calories of food). Look for the following sources of potassium in your diet: raisins, apricots, citrus, pears, melons, bananas, strawberries, cabbage, spinach, peas, parsley, broccoli, peppers, carrots, potato skins, whole grains, turkey, fish, and beef.

Omega-3 Fatty Acids

Omega-3 fatty acids, which represent one of the two classes of polyunsaturated fats, are particularly heart-protective. To help you isolate the foods that contain omega-3s, we've decided to list them separately in the counter. It's estimated that as much as 99 percent of Americans don't consume enough omega-3s, which are obtained either from plant sources (such as flaxseed, walnut, and canola oils, and spinach) or fish (the coldwater variety, such as salmon). Experts tell us we should be getting 1 gram each of plant-derived and marine-derived omega-3s every day. However, if you're using the recommended oils *and* eating the recommended fish at least 2 to 4 times a week, you're certain to benefit from these helpful fats.

Since omega-3 fatty acids are found only in very specific foods, the counter affords them a value of "high" or "na" (not available/ not applicable) in its "Food Descriptions and Nutrients" section. There is no recommended daily intake for omega-3 fatty acids, but do try to incorporate some coldwater fish into your diet at least twice per week.

Sodium

Too much dietary sodium can cause blood pressure levels to rise, increasing your risk for heart disease. The National Heart, Lung, and Blood Institute recommends limiting your sodium intake to no more than

2,400 milligrams per day (the equivalent of about 1 teaspoon of salt)—and less if you can manage it or if you're already suffering from high blood pressure.

When tracking foods in the counter you'll quickly see why processed food is the real culprit when it comes to sodium, which is measured in milligrams (mg) herein. But don't forget about the plethora of reduced-salt or no-salt-added products now available at most supermarkets. And as always, go fresh (rather than frozen, canned, smoked, pickled, cured, or processed) wherever possible.

ABBREVIATIONS AND SYMBOLS

When you look up a food in the nutrition counter, you'll need to understand what the following abbreviations and symbols mean.

Measurements

fl. oz.	fluid ounce
gm	gram
mcg	microgram
mg	milligram
oz.	ounce
tbsp.	tablespoon
tsp.	teaspoon
t	trace
w	with
w/o	without
+	some trans fat
++	high in trans fats

Food Descriptions and Nutrients

0	zero (no nutrient value)
AC	alpha-carotene
BC	beta-carotene
BCR	beta-cryptoxanthin
Sat. Fat	saturated fat
Fat/ Poly.	polyunsaturated fat
Fat/ Mono.	monounsaturated fat
LU+Z	lutein and zeaxanthin
LYC	lycopene
Na or Un	information not available or unknown *(Note: Don't take a designation of "na" or "un" to mean the absence of a particular nutrient, only that analysis of that food for that nutrient is lacking, altogether absent, or present in such minute quantities that they are not applicable here.)*
*SOL	high in soluble fiber

All the information in the Heart-Healthy counter is based on data from the United States government, from brand-name food manufacturers, and from fast-food restaurants and chains. Also consulted were the U.S. Department of Agriculture (USDA) National Nutrient Database, numerous journal articles that analyzed the nutrient content of various foods, and various computer- and Internet-based sources, including Diet Expert, FoodCount.com, and Nutribase.

This counter arms you with everything you need to adopt and maintain a heart-healthy diet—which, as you know now, is also the *sensible* diet nutritionists have been busy promoting for decades. Take it with you wherever you feel it may come in handy. In no time you'll be planning, preparing, and *enjoying* the abundance of foods that truly maximize heart health.

For life.

Food	Serving Size	Calories	Fat/Sat. Fat (gm)	Poly/Mono Fat (gm)	Fiber (gm)	Sugars (gm)	Carotenoids (mcg or mg)	Potassium (mg)	*Omega-3 Fat	Trans Fat	Sodium
BEEF											
**Brisket, braised	3 oz.	185	8.6/3	.3/3.4	0	0	0	928	na	0	44
**Chuck roast, baked	3 oz.	250	16/6	.6/7	0	0	0	207	na	0	58
Chipped, dried	1 slice	15	4/.1	na	0	0	0	na	na	0	na
Corned beef, canned	1 slice	52.5	3/1.3	.13/1.2	0	0	0	29	na	0	211
**Eye of the round	3 oz.	165	7/2.6	.3/3.7	0	0	0	68	na	0	49
**Flank steak	3 oz.	176	8.6/3.7	.3/3	0	0	0	na	na	0	54
Hamburger:											
Beef patty, cooked from frozen	3 oz. (1 patty)	240	17/6.5	2.5/.27	0	0	0	248	na	0	55
Extra lean, broiled medium	3 oz.	218	14/5.5	na	0	0	0	390	na	0	61
Extra lean, broiled well done	3 oz.	225	13.4/5	na	0	0	0	305	na	0	64
Lean, broiled medium	3 oz.	231	16/6	na	0	0	0	289	na	0	69
Lean, broiled well done	3 oz.	238	15/6	.62/7.3	0	0	0	na	na	0	na
Regular, broiled medium	3 oz.	246	17.5/7	na	0	0	0	250	na	0	65
Regular, broiled well done	3 oz.	248	16.5/6.5	na	0	0	0	na	na	0	na

*Counted as "high" or "na"
**Trimmed to 1/8" fat, all grades

107

Food	Serving Size	Calories	Fat/Sat. Fat (gm)	Poly/Mono Fat (gm)	Fiber (gm)	Sugars (gm)	Carotenoids (mcg or mg)	Potassium (mg)	*Omega-3 Fat	Trans Fat	Sodium
**Porterhouse steak, broiled	3 oz.	254	19/7	.7/8	0	0	0	320	na	0	54
Rib-eye steak, broiled	3 oz.	188	10/3.7	na	0	0	0	322	na	0	na
**Round tip, roasted	3 oz.	186	9.6/3.6	.3/3	0	0	0	205	na	0	35
**T-bone steak, broiled	3 oz.	238	16.5/6.4	.6/7	0	0	0	320	na	0	56
**Sirloin steak, broiled	3 oz.	211	12/5	.4/6	0	0	0	286	na	0	62
**Tenderloin, roasted	3 oz.	239	16/6	.8/8.7	0	0	0	331	na	0	48
Variety meats:											
Brain, panfried	3 oz.	167	13.5/3	2/3	0	0	0	304	na	0	134
Heart, simmered	3 oz.	149	5/1.4	.8/.8	0	0	0	186	na	0	50
Liver, panfried	3 oz.	185	7/2.3	.6/.6	0	0	0	284	na	0	77
Tongue, baked	3 oz.	237	17/7.5	.6/8.5	0	0	0	165	na	0	55
BEVERAGES/ALCOHOLIC/BEER											
Beer, light	12 fl. oz.	99	0/0	0/0	0	.32	0	74	na	0	14
Beer, nonalcoholic	12 fl. oz.	216	.4/.1	na	0	na	0	na	na	0	na
Beer, regular	12 fl. oz.	146	0/0	0/0	.7	0	0	96	na	0	14
BEVERAGES/ALCOHOLIC/DISTILLED LIQUORS											
80 proof	1 fl. oz.	64	0/0	0/0	0	0	0	2	na	0	0
90 proof	1 fl. oz.	70	0/0	0/0	0	0	0	1	na	0	0
100 proof	1 fl. oz.	82	0/0	0/0	0	0	0	1	na	0	0

**Trimmed to 1/8" fat, all grades

Food	Serving Size	Calories	Fat/Sat. Fat (gm)	Poly/Mono Fat (gm)	Fiber (gm)	Sugars (gm)	Carotenoids (mcg or mg)	Potassium (mg)	*Omega-3 Fat	Trans Fat	Sodium
BEVERAGES/ALCOHOLIC/WINE											
Champagne	1 wine glass (3.5 fl. oz.)	72	0/0	0/0	0	na	0	na	na	0	na
Dessert, dry	1 wine glass (3.5 fl. oz.)	130	0/0	0/0	0	1.12	0	95	na	0	9
Dessert, sweet	1 wine glass (3.5 fl. oz.)	158	0/0	0/0	0	8	0	95	na	0	9
Nonalcoholic	1 wine glass (3.5 fl. oz.)	6	0/0	0/0	0	1.12	0	89	na	0	7
Red	1 wine glass (3.5 fl. oz.)	74	0/0	0/0	0	1.7	0	115	na	0	5
Rose	1 wine glass (3.5 fl. oz.)	73	0/0	0/0	0	1.4	0	102	na	0	5
Sherry	1 wine glass (3.5 fl. oz.)	158	0/0	0/0	0	na	0	na	na	0	na
White	1 wine glass (3.5 fl. oz.)	70	0/0	0/0	0	.82	0	82	na	0	5
Wine cooler	1 drink (7 fl. oz.)	105	0/0	0/0	.1	na	1.8 mcg (BC)	na	na	0	na
BEVERAGES/COFFEE											
Brewed, decaf	1 cup	4.7	0/0	0	0	0	0	128	na	0	5
Brewed, regular	1 cup	4.7	0/0	0	0	0	0	116	na	0	5
instant, decaf	1 cup	3.5	0/0	0	0	0	0	63	na	0	2
instant, regular	1 cup	3.6	0/0	0	0	0	0	53	na	0	1

Food	Serving Size	Calories	Fat/Sat. Fat (gm)	Poly/Mono Fat (gm)	Fiber (gm)	Sugars (gm)	Carotenoids (mcg or mg)	Potassium (mg)	*Omega-3 Fat	Trans Fat	Sodium
BEVERAGES/FRUIT JUICES											
Acerola juice	1 cup	56	.7/.16	2/.2	.7	10.89	740 mcg	235	Na	0	7
Apple juice, canned, no sugar, w/ added Vit. C	1 cup	117	.27/.04	.08/.01	.25	na	0	119	na	0	7
Apple juice, canned, no sugar, no added Vit. C	1 cup	117	.27/.05	.08/.01	.25	10.9	0	119	na	0	7
Apple juice, concentrate, no sugar, w/ added Vit. C	1 cup	112	.24/.04	.07/t	.24	27.6	0	301	na	0	7
Apple juice, concentrate, no sugar, no added Vit. C	1 cup	112	.24/.04	.07/t	.24	27.6	0	301	na	0	7
Apricot nectar, w/ added Vit. C	1 cup	140.5	.23/.01	na	1.5	36	2 mg (BC)	286	na	0	na
Apricot nectar, no added Vit. C	1 cup	140.5	.23/.01	na	1.5	34.6	2 mg (BC)	286	na	0	na
Grape juice, concentrate, w/added sugar, Vit. C	1 cup	127.5	.23/.07	.7/t	.25	26.12	15 mcg (BC)	53	na	0	17

Food	Serving Size	Calories	Fat/Sat. Fat (gm)	Poly/Mono Fat (gm)	Fiber (gm)	Sugars (gm)	Carotenoids (mcg or mg)	Potassium (mg)	*Omega-3 Fat	Trans Fat	Sodium
Grape juice, unsweetened, w/added Vit. C	1 cup	152	.2/.1	na	.25	na	15 mcg (BC)	na	na	0	na
Grape juice, unsweetened, w/o added Vit. C	1 cup	154	.2/.06	.05/.03	.25	37.6	15 mcg (BC)	334	na	0	8
Grapefruit juice, pink, fresh	1 cup	93	.25/.03	.05/.03	na	22.7	15 mcg (BC)	400	na	0	2
Grapefruit juice, white, fresh	1 cup	96	.25/.03	.05/.03	.25	22.5	15 mcg (BC)	400	na	0	2
Grapefruit juice, sweetened, canned	1 cup	115	.22/.03	.05/.03	.25	27.57	0	405	na	0	5
Grapefruit juice, unsweetened, canned	1 cup	94	.25/.03	.05/.03	.25	21.88	15 mcg (BC)	378	na	0	2
Grapefruit juice, concentrate, sweetened	1 cup	118	.25/t	na	.25	na	12 mcg (BC)	na	na	0	na
Grapefruit juice, concentrate, unsweetened	1 cup	101	.32/.05	.07/.04	.25	23.79	13 mcg (BC)	336	na	0	2
Lemon juice, bottled	1 tbsp.	13	.04/t	.01/t	.06	.36	1.8 mcg (BC)	15	na	0	3
Lemon juice, from 1 lemon	1 fruit	12	0/0	0/0	.19	1.13	7 mcg (BC)	58	na	0	0

111

Food	Serving Size	Calories	Fat/Sat. Fat (gm)	Poly/Mono Fat (gm)	Fiber (gm)	Sugars (gm)	Carotenoids (mcg or mg)	Potassium (mg)	*Omega-3 Fat	Trans Fat	Sodium
Lime juice, bottled	1 tbsp.	3.2	.04/t	.01/t	.06	.21	1.8 mcg (BC)	12	na	0	2
Lime juice, from 1 lime	1 fruit					.64	2 mcg (BC)	44	na	0	1
Mango nectar, canned	1 cup	146	.3/.1	t/t	1.8	31	1.7 mg (BC)	na	na	0	0
Orange juice, fresh	1 cup	112	.5/.06	.09/.09	.5	20.8	298 mcg (BC)	496	na	0	2
Orange juice, canned, unsweetened	1 cup	105	.35/.04	.08/.06	.5	20.9	269 mcg (BC)	436	na	0	5
Orange juice, from carton, unsweetened	1 cup	109.5	0/0		.5	169	269 mcg (BC)	320	na	0	0
Orange juice, from concentrate, diluted	1 cup	112	.15/.01	.03/.02	.5	20.9	119 mcg (BC)	473	na	0	2
Orange-grapefruit, canned, unsweetened	1 cup	106	.25/.03	.03/.02	2.5	20.9	178 mcg (BC)	390	na	0	2
Passion fruit, carton	1 cup	152	0/0	0/0	na	36	165 mcg (BC)	60	na	0	62
Peach nectar, canned, w/ added Vit.C	1 cup	134	.05/t	t/t	1.5	34.7	388 mcg (BC)	100	na	0	na
Peach nectar, canned, w/o added Vit. C	1 cup	134	.05/t	t/t	1.5	34.7	388 mcg (BC)	100	na	0	na

Food	Serving Size	Calories	Fat/Sat. Fat (gm)	Poly/Mono Fat (gm)	Fiber (gm)	Sugars (gm)	Carotenoids (mcg or mg)	Potassium (mg)	*Omega-3 Fat	Trans Fat	Sodium
Pineapple, unsweetened, w/ added Vit. C	1 cup	140	.2/.01	.07/.02	.5	33.95	0	335	na	0	3
Pineapple, unsweetened	1 cup	140	.2/.01	.07/.02	.5	33.95	0	335	na	0	3
Pineapple, from concentrate	1 cup	130	.07/t	.02/t	.5	31.4	0	340	na	0	3
Orange-grapefruit juice	1 cup	80	0/0	0/0	.4	19	8 mcg (BC)	30	na	0	0
Pineapple-orange juice, canned	1 cup	125	0/0	0/0	.25	29	135 mcg (BC)	115	na	0	8
Tropical blend, carton	1 cup	120	0/0	0/0	0	22	68 mcg (BC)	na	na	0	15
Prune juice, bottled or canned	1 cup	182	.07/t	.08/.05	2.6	42.1	0	707	na	0	10
Strawberry-banana-orange juice, carton	1 cup	126	0/0	0/0	2.6	27	28 mcg (BC)	286	na	0	14
BEVERAGES/JUICE DRINKS & PUNCHES											
Cranberry apple drink, bottled	1 cup	165	0/0	0/0	.24	44.1	0	69	na	0	17
Cranberry grape drink, bottled	1 cup	137	.25/.08	.05/.01	.24	34.3	28 mcg (BC)	59	na	0	7

113

Food	Serving Size	Calories	Fat/Sat. Fat (gm)	Poly/Mono Fat (gm)	Fiber (gm)	Sugars (gm)	Carotenoids (mcg or mg)	Potassium (mg)	*Omega-3 Fat	Trans Fat	Sodium
Cranberry juice cocktail, bottled	1 cup	144	.25/.02	.11/.03	.25	34.2	0	46	na	0	5
Cranberry juice cocktail, low-calorie, bottled	1 cup	45	0/0	0/0	0	10.9	0	59	na	0	7
Fruit punch drink, frozen or canned (Hi-C)	1 cup	116	0/0	0/0	.2	28.8	15 mcg (BC)	32	na	0	10
Grape juice drink, canned	1 cup	125	0/0	0/0	.25	31.9	0	na	na	0	3
Kool-Aid, with sugar, prepared, w/ added Vit. C	1 cup	88	0/0	0/0	0	22	1.2 mcg (BC)	0	na	0	20
Crystal Light, low-calorie, prepared	1 cup	43	0/0	0/0	0	.21	14 mcg (BC)	0	na	0	127
Lemonade, from concentrate, diluted	1 cup	99	0/0	0/0	0	25.9	33 mcg (BC)	37	na	0	7
Limeade, from concentrate, diluted	1 cup	101	0/0	0/0	.25	22.1	0	22	na	0	5
Tang Instant Juice Drink, prepared with water, w/ added Vit. C	1 cup	119	0/0	0/0	0	13	0	na	na	0	na
Splash, all flavors (Campbell's)	1 cup	267	.1/0	0/0	.7	na	3 mg (BC)	na	na	0	na

114

Food	Serving Size	Calories	Fat/Sat. Fat (gm)	Poly/Mono Fat (gm)	Fiber (gm)	Sugars (gm)	Carotenoids (mcg or mg)	Potassium (mg)	*Omega-3 Fat	Trans Fat	Sodium
Splash, diet, all flavors (Campbell's)	1 cup	19	0/0	0/0	0	na	na	na	na	0	na
Sports drinks:											
Gatorade (Quaker Oats)	1 cup	60	0/0	0/0	0	14.3	0	32	na	0	96
Gatorade Light (Quaker Oats)	1 cup	26	0/0	0/0	0	na	0	na	na	0	na
BEVERAGES/VEGETABLE JUICES											
Carrot juice, canned	1 cup	94	.35/.06	.16/.01	1.8	9.23	3.6 mg (BC)	689	na	0	68
Tomato juice	1 cup	41	.15/.02	.05/.02	1	8.65	816 mcg–1 mg (BC) 149 mcg (LU+Z)	654	na	0	654
Tomato juice, low sodium	1 cup	41	.15/.02	.1/.03	2	9.2	23 mg (LYC)	169	na	0	169
Tomato juice, with clam juice	1 cup	35	.2/.1	0/0	.7	2.5	816 mcg–1 mg (BC) 23 mg (LYC)	273	na	0	273
Vegetable juice with tomato, low sodium	1 cup	46	.2/.03	.1/.03	2	9.2	520 mcg (AC) 1.7 mg–2 mg (BC) 198 mcg (LU+Z) 24 mg (LYC)	169	na	0	169

Food	Serving Size	Calories	Fat/Sat. Fat (gm)	Poly/Mono Fat (gm)	Fiber (gm)	Sugars (gm)	Carotenoids (mcg or mg)	Potassium (mg)	*Omega-3 Fat	Trans Fat	Sodium
BEVERAGES/NON-MILK, GRAIN BASED											
Cereal grain beverage (Kaffree Roma)	1 cup	6	0/0	0/0	0	.14	na	74	na	0	7
Rice beverage, canned (Rice Dream)	1 cup	120	2/2	.3/1.3	0	72	na	16	na	0	86
Rice beverage original (So Nice)	1 cup	120	3/.8	1.6/.6	0	5	na	250	na	0	130
Rice beverage w/soy (Silk)	1 cup	90	4/.6	.6/.24	0	6	na	300	na	0	120
BEVERAGES/TEA											
Green tea, brewed	1 cup	2.4	0/0	0/0	0	na	0	na	na	0	na
Herbal tea, brewed	1 cup	2.3	0/0	t/t	0	.47	0	21	na	0	2
Iced tea, with lemon (Nestle)	1 cup	88	.7/.05	0/0	0	18	na	na	na	0	0
Tea (black), brewed	1 cup	2.4	0/0	0/0	0	0	0	88	na	0	7
Tea, instant, sweetened, w/added Vit. C	1 cup	88	t/t	.02/t	0	177.6	0	395	na	0	8
BREADS, MUFFINS & ROLLS											
Bagels: Blueberry, refrigerated (Lenders)	1 bagel	209	1.3/.3	.4/.3	2	7.99	t	158	na	0	409

Food	Serving Size	Calories	Fat/Sat. Fat (gm)	Poly/Mono Fat (gm)	Fiber (gm)	Sugars (gm)	Carotenoids (mcg or mg)	Potassium (mg)	*Omega-3 Fat	Trans Fat	Sodium
Cinnamon raisin	1 bagel, 3" dia.	156	1/.15	.38/.1	1.3	3.4	0	84	na	0	183
Egg	1 bagel, 3" dia.	192	1.2/.2	.4/.29	1.3	36.6	na	66	na	0	348
Multigrain	1 bagel, 3" dia.	148	3.5/.5	2/.8	4	8	t	160	high	0	430
Oat bran	1 bagel, 3" dia.	145	.7/.1	.27/.1	2*SOL	.93	0	66	high	0	289
Plain, enriched	1 bagel, 3" dia.	157	1/.12	.39	1.3	.55	0	58	na	0	304
Whole wheat	1 bagel, 3" dia.	151	2.5/.5	1/.9	5.3	7	0	150	high	0	630
Biscuits:											
From home recipe	1 biscuit, 2½" dia	212	16/4	4/7	.9	45	0	122	na	++	586
From mix	1 biscuit, 3" dia.	191	7/1.6	2.4/2.4	1	27.4	0	107	na	+	554
From refrigerated dough	1 biscuit, 2½" dia.	95	4/1	.5/2	.5	105	0	42	na	+	332
From refrigerated dough, low fat	1 biscuit, 2" dia.	59	1/.25	.16/.57	.37	.04	0	39	na	0	300
Bread crumbs	½ cup	395	5.7/1.2	2.2/1	2.4	6.7	0	212	na	un	791

Food	Serving Size	Calories	Fat/Sat. Fat (gm)	Poly/Mono Fat (gm)	Fiber (gm)	Sugars (gm)	Carotenoids (mcg or mg)	Potassium (mg)	*Omega-3 Fat	Trans Fat	Sodium
Bread sticks	1 stick, 7⅞" x ⅜"	41	1/.14	.36/.36	.3	.13	0	12	na	0	66
Bread stuffing	½ cup	178	8.6/1.7	2.6	3	2.1	0	74	na	++	543
Bread stuffing, cornbread	½ cup	179	9/1.8	3.8	3	21.9	52 mcg (BC)	62	na	++	455
Breads:											
Boston brown, canned	1 slice	88	.7/.13	.25/.09	2	5.36	na	140	na	0	284
Branola	1 slice	89	1.2/.3	na	1.4	na	0	na	na	0	na
Cinnamon	1 slice	69	.9/.1	na	.6	na	0	na	na	0	na
Cracked wheat	1 slice	65	1/.23	.2/.57	1.4	14.8	0	53	na	0	161
Egg	1 slice	115	2.4/.3	4.4/.4	1	.71	0	46	na	+	197
French or Vienna	1 medium slice	68.5	.75/.16	.4/.77	.75	.15	0	72	na	0	390
Fruit and nut	1 slice	217	10/2	na	1	na	8.4 mcg (BC)	na	high	0	na
Garlic	1 medium slice	96	3.8/.7	na	.8	na	31 mcg (BC)	na	na	0	na
Granola	1 slice	89	1.2/.3	na	1.4	na	0	na	na	0	na
High fiber, reduced calorie	1 slice	60	.7/.2	na	3	na	0	na	na	0	na
High protein	1 slice	64	.6/.1	na	.8	.27	0	61	na	0	104
Italian	1 medium slice	54	.7/.17	.27/.16	.5	.17	0	22	na	0	117
Low gluten	1 slice	73	1.4/.2	na	1.5	na	0	44	na	0	na

118

Food	Serving Size	Calories	Fav/Sat. Fat (gm)	Poly/Mono Fat (gm)	Fiber (gm)	Sugars (gm)	Carotenoids (mcg or mg)	Potassium (mg)	*Omega-3 Fat	Trans Fat	Sodium
Mixed grain (7-grain, whole grain)	1 slice	65	1/.2	.25/1	1.7	na	0	na	high	0	na
Mixed grain, reduced calorie	1 slice	52.5	.6/1	na	3	na	0	na	high	0	122
Oat bran	1 slice	71	1.3/.2	.5/.47	1.3*SOL	2.31	0	44	na	0	na
Oat bran, reduced calorie	1 slice	46	.7/.1	.38/15	2.7*SOL	.81	0	23	na	0	81
Oatmeal	1 slice	72	1.2/.4	.46/42	1	2.2	0	38	na	0	162
Oatmeal, reduced calorie	1 slice	48	.8/.14	.3/.18	na	43.3	0	124	na	0	89
Prairie Bran	2 slices	220	3/5	1/5	2*SOL	4	0	na	na	0	470
Pita, white, enriched	1 large, 6.5" dia.	165	.72/.1	.3/.06	1.3	.78	0	na	na	0	322
Pita, whole wheat	1 large, 6.5" dia.	170	1.7/.3	.67/2	5	.5	0	72	na	0	340
Potato	1 slice	69	.9/1	na	.6	na	0	na	na	0	na
Pumpernickel	1 slice	50	.6/.08	.3/.2	1.3	.14	0	54	na	0	174
Pumpernickel, marbled with rye	1 slice	66	.8/1	na	1.6	na	0	na	na	0	na
Raisin	1 slice	71	1.1/.3	.17/.59	1	5.7	0	59	na	0	101
Rice bran	1 slice	66	1.2/.5	.47/.44	1.3	1.26	0	58	na	0	119
Rye, light or dark	1 slice	52	1.6/.2	.2/4	1.2	.08	0	53	na	0	211
Rye, reduced calorie	1 slice	46	.6/.08	.17/15	3	.53	0	23	na	0	93

Food	Serving Size	Calories	Fat/Sat. Fat (gm)	Poly/Mono Fat (gm)	Fiber (gm)	Sugars (gm)	Carotenoids (mcg or mg)	Potassium (mg)	*Omega-3 Fat	Trans Fat	Sodium
Rye, snack-sized	1 slice	18	.23/.04	.05/.09	.4	.02	0	46	na	0	46
Sprouted grain, inc. Ezekiel bread	1 slice	65	1/2	na	1	na		na	na	0	na
Sunflower Flax	2 slices	250	5/1	3/1	4*SOL 6	na	na	na	high	0	na
Sweet potato	1 slice	74	1.6/.3	na	.5	na	190 mcg (BC)	na	na	0	na
Sunflower seed	1 slice	75	1.4/.4	na	1.6	na	2 mcg (BC)	na	high	0	na
Triticale	1 slice	63	1/2	na	1	na	0	na	na	0	na
Wheat, including wheatberry	1 slice	65	1/2	.22/.43	2.8	1.37	0	50	na	0	133
Wheat, reduced calorie	1 slice	45	.5/.07	.22/.05	.6	.71	0	28	na	0	118
Wheat germ	1 slice	73	.8/.2	.18/.35	.6	1.04	0	71	high	0	155
White, enriched	2 slices	151	1.8/.3	.8/.4	.8	28	0	na	na	0	na
White, from recipe with 2% milk	1 slice	120	2.4/.5	1/.5	na	20.8	0	61	na	0	151
White, reduced calorie	1 slice	48	.6/.12	.12/.24	2.2	1.09	0	17	na	0	104
Whole wheat	1 slice	69	1.2/.25	.28/.47	2	5.56	0	71	na	0	148
Whole wheat, prepared from recipe	1 slice	128	2.5/.36	1.3/.5	2.8	1.77	0	144	na	0	159
Whole Wheat Soy	2 slices	240	3.5/1	na	4	na	na	300	high	0	450

Food	Serving Size	Calories	Fat/Sat. Fat (gm)	Poly/Mono Fat (gm)	Fiber (gm)	Sugars (gm)	Carotenoids (mcg or mg)	Potassium (mg)	*Omega-3 Fat	Trans Fat	Sodium
Cornbread:											
Prepared from recipe, with 2% milk	1 piece	188	6/1.6	2/1	1.4	28	38 mcg (BC)	96	na	0	428
Prepared from mix	1 piece	140	4.5/1.5	.7/3	2	28.8	20 mcg (BC)	77	na	0	467
Croissant	1 medium	231	12/6.6	.6/3	1.5	6.42	46 mcg (BC)	67	na	++	424
Croutons, plain	½ cup	61	1/23	.19/.45	.75	11	0	67	na	0	105
English muffins:											
Mixed grain	1 muffin	155	1/1.5	.36/.54	2	na	0	103	high	0	275
Plain, enriched	1 muffin	134	1/1.5	.46/.17	1.5	1.68	0	131	na	0	265
Raisin	1 muffin	138.5	1.5/.23	.78/.29	1.7	11.3	0	119	na	0	255
Wheat	1 muffin	127	1/.16	.47/.16	2.6	.89	0	106	na	0	218
Whole wheat	1 muffin	134	1.4/.2	.55/.33	4.4	5.34	0	139	na	0	420
Muffins, commercially prepared:											
Blueberry	1 muffin	183	4.2/.9	1.6/1.3	1.5	13	10 mcg (BC)	81	na	un	259
Bran	1 muffin	168	5/.8	2.7/1.1	4.4*SOL	5.44	0	na	na	un	na
Carrot	1 muffin	174	6.6/.9	na	1	na	1.4 mg (BC)	na	na	un	na
Cheese	1 muffin	177	7/.2	na	.7	na	13 mcg (BC)	na	na	un	344
Corn	1 muffin	160.5	5/1.4	2.1/1.3	1.2	11.73	0	78	na	un	259
Oat bran	1 muffin	154	4/.6	2.7/1.1	2.6*SOL	5.4	0	na	573	un	na
Oatmeal	1 muffin	136	3.5/.9	na	.8*SOL	na	2.4 mcg (BC)	na	na	un	na
Plain	1 muffin	175	6/1.5	na	.7	na	3 mcg (BC)	na	na	un	na
Pumpkin	1 muffin	178	4/.7	na	1	na	1.9 mg (BC)	na	na	un	na

Food	Serving Size	Calories	Fat/Sat. Fat (gm)	Poly/Mono Fat (gm)	Fiber (gm)	Sugars (gm)	Carotenoids (mcg or mg)	Potassium (mg)	*Omega-3 Fat	Trans Fat	Sodium
Toaster muffin	1 muffin	110	3.3/.5	1.7/.73	.6	7.8	1.8 mcg (BC)	30	na	un	78
Zucchini	1 muffin	215	11/1.5	na	.8	na	26 mcg (BC)	na	na	un	na
Muffins, from home recipe:											
Blueberry (with 2% milk)	1 muffin	162	6/1	3.1/.4	na	23	10 mcg (BC)	70	na	un	251
Bran	1 muffin	168	5/.8	na	4.4*SOL	na	0	na	na	un	na
Corn	1 muffin	180	7/1.3	3.5/1.7	na	25.2	na	145	na	un	333
Plain	1 muffin	169	6.5/1.3	3.2/1.5	1.5	23.6	0	69	na	un	26
Muffins, toaster:											
Blueberry	1 muffin	103	3/.5	1.7/.7	.6	3.97	na	27	na	0	158
Corn	1 muffin	114	4/.5	2/.86	.5	19.1	na	31	na	0	142
Wheat bran	1 muffin	106	3/.5	1.7/.73	3*SOL	18.8	na	60	na	0	178
Rolls and buns:											
Cloverleaf	1 roll	103	1.8/.4	na	1	na	0	na	na	0	na
Dinner roll, egg	1 roll, 2½" dia.	107.5	2/.5	.39/1	1.3	1.6	0	36	na	0	191
Dinner roll, plain	1 roll	85	2/.5	.33/1	.9	1.6	0	37	na	0	146
Dinner roll, rye	1 small, 2½" dia.	81	1/.17	.19/.34	1.4	.33	0	50	na	0	250
Dinner roll, wheat	1 roll	77	1.8/.4	.31/.87	1	.46	0	32	na	0	95
Dinner roll, whole wheat	1 roll, 2½" dia.	96	1.7/.3	.77/.43	2.7	3.05	0	98	na	0	172
French roll	1 roll	105	1.6/.36	.31/.74	1	.12	0	43	na	0	231
Hamburger bun, whole wheat, large	1 bun	206	2.6/.8	.7/.7	1.6	3.6	0	212	na	0	442

122

Food	Serving Size	Calories	Fat/Sat. Fat (gm)	Poly/Mono Fat (gm)	Fiber (gm)	Sugers (gm)	Carotenoids (mcg or mg)	Potassium (mg)	*Omega-3 Fat	Trans Fat	Sodium
Hamburger bun, plain	1 bun	123	2/.5	.8/.4	1	2	0	60	na	0	300
Hamburger bun, whole wheat flax, large	1 roll, 8" dia.	202	7.3/1.2	1.1/3.5	3.3	29	0	na	high	0	na
Hotdog bun, whole wheat, large	1 bun	234	3/.8	.8/.9	1.6	4	0	na	na	0	504
Hotdog bun, plain	1 bun	140	1.5/.4	.8/.3	1	2	0	65	na	0	290
Submarine/hoagie bun	1 bun, 8" long	269	5/1	na	2.5	na	0	na	na	0	na
Tacos:											
Corn, large	1 taco, 6½" dia.	98	4.7/.7	na	1.6	na	0	na	na	+	na
Corn, medium	1 taco, 5" dia.	62	3/.4	na	1	19	0	na	na	+	na
Flour, large	1 taco, 10" dia.	286	15/3.6	na	2	34	0	na	na	+	na
Flour, regular	1 taco, 7" dia.	173.5	9/2.2	na	1	31	0	na	na	+	na
Tortillas:											
Corn, large	1 tortilla, 8" dia.	73	.8/.1	na	1.7	na	0	na	na	0	na
Corn, medium	1 tortilla, 6" dia.	42	.5/.1	na	1	na	0	na	na	0	na

123

Food	Serving Size	Calories	Fat/Sat. Fat (gm)	Poly/Mono Fat (gm)	Fiber (gm)	Sugars (gm)	Carotenoids (mcg or mg)	Potassium (mg)	*Omega-3 Fat	Trans Fat	Sodium
Flour, large	1 tortilla, 10" dia.	218	5/1.2	na	2	na	0	na	na	+	na
Flour, medium	1 tortilla, 8" dia.	140	3/.8	na	1.4	na	0	na	na	+	na
Whole wheat, large	1 tortilla, 8" dia	109	.7/.1	na	3	na	0	na	na	0	na
Whole wheat, medium	1 tortilla, 7" dia.	103	3.1/.65	1.2/.7	3.3	29	0	na	na	0	na

CAKES/PIES, LOWFAT

Food	Serving Size	Calories	Fat/Sat. Fat (gm)	Poly/Mono Fat (gm)	Fiber (gm)	Sugars (gm)	Carotenoids (mcg or mg)	Potassium (mg)	*Omega-3 Fat	Trans Fat	Sodium
Angel Food Cake (Krogers)	1 slice	150	0/0	na	0	24	na	na	na	0	160
Apple Raisin Spice Cake (Weight Watchers)	1 serving	173	4/.9	na	1.6	na	70 mcg (BC)	na	na	un	165
Brownie, fudge, Lite Bites (Entenmann's)	1 piece	280	15/3.5	na	2	24	0	na	na	un	190
Brownie, Reduced Fat (Little Debbie)	1 serving	190	3/1	na	1	27	0	na	na	un	200
Brownie, Fudge, Fat-Free (No Pudge)	1 serving	110	0/0	na	1	22	na	na	na	0	100

124

Food	Serving Size	Calories	Fat/Sat. Fat (gm)	Poly/Mono Fat (gm)	Fiber (gm)	Sugars (gm)	Carotenoids (mcg or mg)	Potassium (mg)	*Omega-3 Fat	Trans Fat	Sodium
Brownie, Cappuccino, Fat-Free (No Pudge)	1 serving	110	0/0	na	1	22	na	na	na	0	100
Brownie, Raspberry, Fat-Free (No Pudge)	1 serving	110	0/0	na	0	17	na	na	na	0	120
Carrot cake, fat-free (Entenmann's)	1 slice	170	0/0	na	1	na	na	na	na	0	na
Chocolate cake, sugar-free (Sweet n' Low)	1/6 cake	150	3/1	na	1	na	0	na	na	0	na
Coffee cake/Danish, Raspberry, Light (Entenmann's)	1 piece	140	0/0	na	1	199	1.2 mcg (BC)	na	na	0	160
Crumb cake, low fat (Hostess)	1 serving	90	.5/0	na	0	16	0	na	na	0	100
Cupcake, chocolate, w/frosting, low fat	1 cupcake	131	1.6/.5	na	2	na	0	na	na	0	na
Chocolate Éclair, low fat (Weight Watchers)	1 eclair	150	4/1	na	1	13	na	na	na	0	170
Devil's Food Cake, reduced fat (Sweet Rewards)	1 serving	160	1.5/.5	na	1	na	0	na	na	0	na

Food	Serving Size	Calories	Fat/Sat. Fat (gm)	Poly/Mono Fat (gm)	Fiber (gm)	Sugars (gm)	Carotenoids (mcg or mg)	Potassium (mg)	*Omega-3 Fat	Trans Fat	Sodium
Double Fudge Cake (Weight Watchers)	1 serving	190	4.5/1	na	2	na	0	na	na	++	na
Fudge Iced Chocolate cake, nonfat (Entenmann's)	1 slice	210	0/0	na	2	na	0	na	na	0	na
German Chocolate Cake (Weight Watchers)	2.5 oz. serving	200	7/1	na	0	na	0	na	na	++	na
Key Lime Pie (Weight Watchers)	1 slice	200	6/2.5	na	0	24	na	na	na	++	80
Lemon cake, w/icing, low fat (DuncanHines Delights)	1 piece	382	10/2	na	.3	na	44 mcg (BC)	na	na	un	na
Mississippi Mud Pie (Weight Watchers)	1 slice	190	4.5/2	na	1	15	na	na	na	++	120
Peanut Butter Pie (Weight Watchers)	1 slice	210	6/1.5	na	1	14	0	na	na	++	240
Pound cake, fat-free (Entenmann's)	1 piece	150	4/1	na	0	13	0	na	na	0	170
Pound cake, chocolate, fat-free (Entenmann's)	1 slice	79	.3/.1	na	1	na	0	na	na	0	na
Pound cake, reduced fat (Sara Lee Free & Light)	1 slice	77	.3/.1	na	.3	na	na	na	na	0	na

126

Food	Serving Size	Calories	Fat/Sat. Fat (gm)	Poly/Mono Fat (gm)	Fiber (gm)	Sugars (gm)	Carotenoids (mcg or mg)	Potassium (mg)	*Omega-3 Fat	Trans Fat	Sodium
Shortcake Snack (Weight Watchers)	1 serving	170	2/1	na	0	na	0	na	na	0	na
White cake, eggless, low fat	1 piece	165	3.6/.6	na	.4	na	1.2 mcg (BC)	na	na	un	na
CEREALS											
Cold Cereals											
100% Bran (Post)	½ cup	83	.6/.08	0/0	8.3*SOL	7	0	na	na	0	120
100% Natural Oats & Honey (Kellogg's)	½ cup	213	8/3.5	.96/2.3	3.6*SOL	13.3	0	252	na	0	24
All Bran Flakes (Ralston)	1 cup	110	.5/0	na	7*SOL	4	0	180	na	0	290
All Bran Bran Buds (Kellogg's)	½ cup	83	.7/.12	.37/.14	12*SOL	8	0	180	na	0	201
All Bran (Kellogg's)	½ cup	79	.9/.2	.03/.2	9.7*SOL	4.7	0	420	na	0	73
All Bran w/ extra fiber (Kellogg's)	½ cup	53	1/.17	.66/.21	15*SOL	.11	0	na	na	0	143
Almond Delight	½ cup	100	1.5/.4	na	1.5	na	0	na	na	0	na
Alpen	½ cup	199	1.8/.3	.52/.75	5*SOL	11.3	56 mcg (BC)	na	high	0	na
Amaranth Flakes	1 cup	134	4/.8	na	3.6	na	0	na	high	0	120
Apple Raisin Crisps (Kellogg's)	1 cup	185	.5/.1	na	4	na	20 mcg (BC)	na	na	0	na

Food	Serving Size	Calories	Fat/Sat. Fat (gm)	Poly/Mono Fat (gm)	Fiber (gm)	Sugars (gm)	Carotenoids (mcg or mg)	Potassium (mg)	*Omega-3 Fat	Trans Fat	Sodium
Banana Nut Crunch (Post)	1 cup	249	6/8	0/0	4	12	0	171	na	un	253
Basic 4 (General Mills)	1 cup	200	3/.4	na	3.4	na	0	na	na	+	na
Bran Chex (Kellogg's)	1 cup	156	1.4/.2	na	8	na	0	na	na	0	na
Bran Flakes (Kellogg's)	⅔ cup	95	.6/.12	.32/.14	4.6*SOL	4.9	0	120	na	0	207
Bran Flakes (Post)	⅔ cup	233	1/0	na	4.7*SOL	5	6.6 mcg (BC)	na	na	0	170
Cheerios multigrain (General Mills)	1 cup	112	1/.25	.15/.29	2*SOL	6	0	88	high	0	201
Common Sense Oat Bran Flakes (Kellogg's)	¾ cup	109	1/.36	.3/.51	4*SOL	6	0	120	na	0	210
Corn Bran (Quaker)	1 cup	120	1/.3	na	6.4*SOL	10	30 mcg (BC)	na	na	0	250
Corn Chex (Ralston)	1 cup	113	.36/.07	na	.5	3.2	0	25	na	0	288
Corn Flakes	1 cup	102	.2/.05	.09/.03	.8	2.94	0	33	na	0	202
Cracklin Oat Bran (Kellogg's)	¾ cup	225	7/3	1.1/4.5	6.5*SOL	17	0	248	na	0	157
Crispix (Kellogg's)	1 cup	108	.3/.09	.09/.03	.6	2.9	0	na	na	0	202
Crunchy Bran (Ralston)	¾ cup	90	.9/.2	na	5	na	0	na	na	0	na
Fiber One (General Mills)	½ cup	61.5	.8/.13	.41/.13	14*SOL	10	0	232	na	0	129

Food	Serving Size	Calories	Fat/Sat. Fat (gm)	Poly/Mono Fat (gm)	Fiber (gm)	Sugars (gm)	Carotenoids (mcg or mg)	Potassium (mg)	*Omega-3 Fat	Trans Fat	Sodium
Frosted Shredded Wheat (Post)	1 cup	190	1/0	.5/0	6*SOL	11	0	160	na	0	0
Fruit and Fiber (Post)	1 cup	212	3/.4	na	5	na	0	na	na	0	na
Fruit Granola, low fat (Nature's Valley)	¾ cup	212	3/.4	.63/1.6	3.4*SOL	18.5	0	154	high	0	208
Fruit N' Nut Granola (Nature's Valley)	¾ cup	253	11/2	.13/9.3	3.4	na	0	na	na	0	na
Granola, homemade	1 cup	570	30/6	na	13*SOL	24.5	0	655	high	un	27
Granola, low fat (Kellogg's)	½ cup	213	3/.5	.77/1.4	3.2*SOL	15.7	0	166	high	0	135
Grape Nuts (Post)	½ cup	208	5/0	t/t	6*SOL	5	0	na	na	0	170
Grape Nuts Flakes (Post)	¾ cup	106	.8/.17	na	3*SOL	4	0	na	na	0	na
Great Grains Raisin, Date & Pecan (Post)	¾ cup	203	4.5/.6	0/0	4*SOL	13.3	na	177	high	+	156
Heartland Natural	1 cup	500	18/4.5	na	7	na	na	na	na	0	na
Honeybran	1 cup	119	.7/.25	na	4*SOL	na	0	na	na	0	na
Kashi	1 cup	120	.7/.1	.3/.3	4.5	na	0	80	high	0	6
King Vitaman (Quaker)	1¼ cup	120	1/.25	.2/.15	1.2	na	0	na	na	0	na
Kix (General Mills)	1⅓ cup	114	.6/.17	.2/.15	.8	3	0	35	na	0	267
Kretschmer Honey Crunch Wheat Germ 1¾ cup		52	1/.15	na	1.5	3.3	0	na	na	0	na

Food	Serving Size	Calories	Fat/Sat. Fat (gm)	Poly/Mono Fat (gm)	Fiber (gm)	Sugars (gm)	Carotenoids (mcg or mg)	Potassium (mg)	*Omega-3 Fat	Trans Fat	Sodium
Kroger Shredded Wheat	1¼ cup	170	1/0	.5/0	6	1	0	na	na	0	na
Life (Quaker)	1 cup	167	1.8/.3	na	3	6	11 mcg (BC)	na	na	0	na
Mueslix (Kellogg's)	⅔ cup	200	3.2/.4	.99/1.6	3.7	17.13		241	high	0	171
Multi-Bran Chex	1 cup	165	1.2/.2	.53/.29	6.4*SOL	10.8	0	190	na	0	322
Multi-Grain Flakes (Kellogg's)	1 cup	104	.36/.03	na	3	na	0	na	na	0	na
Nutri-Grain (Kellogg's)	⅘ cup	100	1/.06	na	4	na	0	na	na	0	na
Oat Bran Cereal (Quaker)	1¼ cup	213	3/.5	1.1/.89	6*SOL	9.3	0	250	na	0	207
Oat Life (Quaker)	¾ cup	121	1.3/.24	.45/.47	2*SOL	6.2	0	91	na	0	164
Oatmeal Crisp (Quaker)	½ cup	120	1.1/.2	.3/.4	.7*SOL	9	0	96	na	0	139
Product 19 (Kellogg's)	1 cup	110	.4/.03	.21/.12	1	3.9	0	50	na	0	207
Puffed Rice	1 cup	56	.07/.01	0/0	.24	12.6	0	16	na	0	0
Puffed Wheat	1 cup	44	.14/.02	0/0	.5	9.55	0	42	na	0	0
Puffins (Barbara's)	¾ cup	100	1/0	na	6	6	na	45	na	0	150
Raisin Bran (Kellogg's)	1 cup	186	1.5/0	.88/3	8*SOL	19.5	0	372	na	0	362
Raisin Bran (Post)	1 cup	187	1/.17	.59/.26	8*SOL	15.7	0	343	na	0	274
Raisin Nut Bran (General Mills)	1 cup	209	4.4/.7	1.6/.26	5	29	0	238	high	0	455

Food	Serving Size	Calories	Fat/Sat. Fat (gm)	Poly/Mono Fat (gm)	Fiber (gm)	Sugars (gm)	Carotenoids (mcg or mg)	Potassium (mg)	*Omega-3 Fat	Trans Fat	Sodium
Rice Chex (General Mills)	1¼ cup	117	.16/.04	.07/.07	.23	2.5	0	30	na	0	292
Rice Krispies (Kellogg's)	1¼ cup	124	.36/.13	.12/.09	.36	3.66	0	39	na	0	319
Shredded Wheat (Post)	2 biscuits	156	.5/.09	na	5.3	na	0	na	na	0	na
Shredded Wheat, spoon-sized (Post)	1 cup	167	.5/.1	0/0	5.6	.44	0	203	na	0	3
Shredded Wheat and Bran (Post)	1¼ cup	197	.8/.1	0/0	8*SOL	.59	0	248	na	0	3
Smart Start (Kellogg's)	¾ cup	103	.5/.3	.45/.1	1	14	0	90	na	0	275
Special K (Kellogg's)	1 cup	115	.3/0	.25/.12	1	4	0	61	na	0	224
Wheat Chex (Ralston)	1 cup	104	.7/.12	na	3.3	na	0	na	na	0	na
Wheaties (General Mills)	1 cup	110	1/.2	.35/.28	2	4.2	0	111	na	0	218
Hot Cereals											
Corn grits, prepared:											
Instant (butter flavor)	1 packet	102	1.5/.68	.14/.27	2.2	.24	0	41	na	0	367
Regular, white	1 cup	145	.5/.07	.19/.12	.5	31.5	0	53	na	0	540
Regular, yellow	1 cup	145	.5/.07	.2/.1	.5	.24	0	51	na	0	540
Cream of rice	1 cup	127	.24/.05	.06/.07	.25	.05	0	49	na	0	2

131

Food	Serving Size	Calories	Fat/Sat. Fat (gm)	Poly/Mono Fat (gm)	Fiber (gm)	Sugars (gm)	Carotenoids (mcg or mg)	Potassium (mg)	*Omega-3 Fat	Trans Fat	Sodium
Cream of wheat:											
Instant	1 cup	149	.5/.09	.32/.08	1.4	.17	0	49	na	0	10
Regular	1 cup	126	.5/.08	.26/.06	1	.15	0	45	na	0	146
With fruit & maple	1 pkt.	132	.5/.06	0/0	.5	28.9	0	56	na	0	242
Farina	1 cup	116.5	.23/.02	.03/.01	3.3	.09	0	na	na	0	5
Malt-O-Meal	1 cup	171	1/.2	na	2	na	0	30	na	0	na
Multi-Grain (Roman Meal)	1 cup	147	1/.13	na	8	na	0	na	na	0	na
Nutrition for Women, oats & soy (Quaker)	1 packet	160	2/.5	na	3*SOL	15.9	0	na	high	0	316
Oat bran	½ cup	146	3/.6	.2/.04	6*SOL	.57	0	210	na	0	2
Oatmeal:											
Flavored	1 packet	157	2/.36	.62/.75	2.8*SOL	13	0	228	na	0	261
Instant (fortified)	½ cup	64	1/.17	.39/.17	4.5*SOL	13	0	124	na	0	53
Regular (not fortified)	½ cup	74	1.2/1.93	.44/.37	2*SOL	1.7	0	131	na	0	1
Wheatena	1 cup	136	1.2/.2	.61/.17	6.6	na	0	187	na	0	5
CHEESE											
Blue or Roquefort	1 oz.	99	8/5	.23/2.2	0	.14	13 mcg (BC)	73	na	0	395
Brick	1 oz.	105	8.4/5.3	.22/2.4	0	.1	22 mcg (BC)	39	na	0	159
Brie	1 oz.	93	7.8/5	.23/2.3	0	.13	15 mcg (BC)	39	na	0	178
Camembert	1 oz.	84	7/4	.2/2	0	.13	20 mcg (BC)	53	na	0	239
Cheddar	1 oz.	110	9/6	.27/2.7	0	.15	30 mcg (BC)	28	na	0	176
Cheddar, low fat	1 oz.	48	2/1.2	.06/.59	0	.15	6.6 mcg (BC)	19	na	0	174

Food	Serving Size	Calories	Fat/Sat. Fat (gm)	Poly/Mono Fat (gm)	Fiber (gm)	Sugars (gm)	Carotenoids (mcg or mg)	Potassium (mg)	*Omega-3 Fat	Trans Fat	Sodium
Colby	1 oz.	110	9/6	.27/.26	0	.15	30 mcg (BC)	36	na	0	171
Cottage:											
1% fat	½ cup	82	1/.7	.03/.33	0	3.07	na	97	na	0	459
2% fat	½ cup	101	2/1.3	.07/.62	0	.37	na	108	na	0	459
Creamed, large or small curd	½ cup	117	5/3	.15/1.3	0	.3	na	88	na	0	425
Nonfat	½ cup	62	.3/.2	t/t	0	1.3	na	23	na	0	9
With fruit	½ cup	110	4.3/2.6	.14/1.2	0	2.7	6.6 mcg (BC)	102	na	0	389
Cream:											
Low fat	1 tbsp.	35	2.6/1.7	.09/.07	0	.03	11 mcg (BC)	25	na	0	44
Nonfat	1 tbsp.	15	.2/.1	t/.05	0	.06	0	24	na	0	82
Regular	1 tbsp.	51	5/3	.2/.14	0	.03	na	17	na	0	43
Edam or Gouda	1 oz.	100	8/5	.19/2.2	0	.63	18 mcg (BC)	34	na	0	232
Feta	1 oz.	74	6/4	.17/1.3	0	1.16	5 mcg (BC)	18	na	0	316
Gruyere	1 oz.	115	9/5	4.9/2.8	0	.1	55 mcg (BC)	23	na	0	95
Gorgonzola	1 oz.	99	8/5	na	0	na	13 mcg (BC)	na	na	0	na
Limburger	1 oz.	92	7.6/4.7	.14/2.4	0	.14	25 mcg (BC)	36	na	0	na
Monterey Jack	1 oz.	104.5	8.5/5.3	na	0	.6	52 mcg (BC)	na	na	0	227
Monterey Jack, low fat	1 oz.	88	6/4	na	0	.5	0	na	na	0	na
Mozzarella, whole milk	1 oz.	79	6/3.7	.22	0	.29	21.6 mcg (BC)	22	na	0	178
Mozzarella, part skim	1 oz.	78	5/3	1.9	0	.32	17 mcg (BC)	24	na	0	175
Mozzarella, fat-free	1 oz.	42	0/0	.13/.13	0	.44	5 mcg (BC)	32	na	0	223

Food	Serving Size	Calories	Fat/Sat. Fat (gm)	Poly/Mono Fat (gm)	Fiber (gm)	Sugars (gm)	Carotenoids (mcg or mg)	Potassium (mg)	*Omega-3 Fat	Trans Fat	Sodium
Meunster	1 oz.	103	8.4/5.4	0/0	0	na	22 mcg (BC)	na	na	0	na
Parmesan or Romano, dry grated	1 tbsp.	23	1.5/1	.06/.42	0	.04	9.6 mcg (BC)	6	na	0	76
Parmesan or Romano, hard	1 oz.	111	7.3/4.7	.16/2.1	0	.23	44 mcg (BC)	26	na	0	454
Provolone	1 oz.	98	7.5/5	.22/2	0	.16	8.4 mcg (BC)	39	na	0	248
Ricotta:											
Light (Sargento)	¼ cup	60	2.5/1.5	na	0	na	na	na	na	0	na
Low fat (Frigo)	¼ cup	64	2/1	na	0	na	na	na	na	0	na
Nonfat (Frigo)	¼ cup	47.5	.4/.2	na	0	na	na	na	na	0	na
Part-skim	¼ cup	80	5/3	.16/1.4	0	.19	na	77	na	0	77
Whole milk	¼ cup	108	8/5	.24/22	0	.17	na	65	na	0	52
Swiss	1 oz.	105	7.7/5	.29/2.2	0	.4	13 mcg (BC)	22	na	0	58
Swiss, low fat	1 oz.	50	1.4/.9	.05/.4	0	11	13 mcg (BC)	31	na	0	78
CHEESE PRODUCTS											
American cheese, singles	1 oz.	90	4.7/1.5	na	0	2.1	53 mcg (BC)	50	na	0	na
American cheese food, spread, from jar	1 oz.	83	6/4	.18/1.8	0	2.5	39 mcg (BC)	69	na	0	461
American cheese, nonfat	1 slice	31	.2/.15	na	0	1.4	na	na	na	0	273
Cheese food (Velveeta)	1 oz.	80	6/4	na	0	2.3	na	94	na	0	420

134

Food	Serving Size	Calories	Fat/Sat. Fat (gm)	Poly/Mono Fat (gm)	Fiber (gm)	Sugars (gm)	Carotenoids (mcg or mg)	Potassium (mg)	*Omega-3 Fat	Trans Fat	Sodium
Cheese food, reduced fat (Velveeta)	1 oz.	62	3/2	na	0	2.4	na	na	na	0	444
Cheese food, Swiss (Velveeta)	1 oz.	100	7/4	na	0	1.8	na	81	na	0	na
CHICKEN											
Fried, batter dipped:											
Breast	1 breast	218	11/3	2.6/4.6	.25	na	0	169	na	0	231
Drumstick	1 drumstick	115	6.7/1.8	1.6/2.8	.13	3.6	0	80	na	0	116
Thigh	1 thigh	238	14/4	2.03/3.5	.26	4.7	0	100	na	0	150
Wing	1 wing	94	6/1.7	1.5/2.6	.09	3.2	0	40	na	0	93
Fried, flour coated:											
Breast	1 breast	131	5/1.5	1.2/2	.06	.97	0	153	na	0	45
Drumstick	1 drumstick	71	4/1	.94/1.6	.03	.47	0	66	na	0	26
Thigh	1 thigh	162	9/2.5	2.1/.6	.06	1.97	0	34	na	0	55
Wing	1 wing	61	4/1.15	.94/1.7	.02	.45	0	34	na	0	15
Ground:											
Patty, cooked	1 patty (4 oz.)	143	8/2.3	na	0	na	0	na	na	0	na
Roasted:											
Breast (meat only)	1 breast	86	2/.5	.4/.54	0	0	0	133	na	0	38
Breast (meat & skin)	1 breast	114	4.5/1.2	.96/1.7	0	0	0	142	na	0	41
Dark meat	1 cup	269	12.6/3.4	3.2/5	0	0	0	194	na	0	130
Leg	1 leg	109	5/1.3	1.1/1.7	0	0	0	138	na	0	52

Food	Serving Size	Calories	Fat/Sat. Fat (gm)	Poly/Mono Fat (gm)	Fiber (gm)	Sugars (gm)	Carotenoids (mcg or mg)	Potassium (mg)	*Omega-3 Fat	Trans Fat	Sodium
Light meat	1 cup	242	6/1.7	1.4/2.1	0	0	0	330	na	0	108
Thigh	1 thigh	91	6/1.6	1.3/2.1	0	0	0	74	na	0	46
Wing	1 wing	61	4/1.14	.87/1.6	0	0	0	27	na	0	17
Canned, boneless	1 can (5 oz.)	230	10/2.8	2.5/4	0	0	0	191	na	0	169
Giblets:											
Fried	1 cup	402	19.5/5.5	4.9/6.4	0	6.3	0	479	na	0	164
Simmered	1 cup	228	7/2	1.2/1.4	0	0	0	325	na	0	97
Liver:											
Simmered	1 cup	220	7.6/2.6	1.5/1.7	0	0	0	329	na	0	95
CONDIMENTS											
A-1 Steak Sauce	1 tbsp.	18	0/0	na	0	na	89 mcg (BC)	na	na	0	
Au jus gravy, canned	¼ cup	9.5	.12/.06	t/.05	0	1.4	0	48	na	0	30
Au jus gravy mix, prep. as directed	¼ cup	10	0/0	0/0	0	1.5	0	0	na	0	348
Barbecue sauce	1 tbsp.	15	2/0	.1/.1	.1	1.25	83 mcg (BC)	16	na	0	122
Bearnaise sauce	1 packet	91	2.2/.3	.8/.3	0	14.9	na	73	na	0	848
Beef gravy, canned	¼ cup	31	1.4/.7	.05/.56	.23	.01	0	47	na	0	326
Beef gravy, nonfat	¼ cup	15	0/0	na	0	na	0	na	na	0	na
Brown gravy, canned or jar	¼ cup	25	1/0	.03/.25	0	.3	0	na	na	0	335
Brown gravy mix, prep. w/water	¼ cup	16	0/0	na	0	na	0	na	na	0	na
Catsup	1 tbsp.	15	.07/.01	.03/.01	0	3.3	91 mcg (BC) 2.6 mg (LYC)	57	na	0	167

Food	Serving Size	Calories	Fat/Sat. Fat (gm)	Poly/Mono Fat (gm)	Fiber (gm)	Sugars (gm)	Carotenoids (mcg or mg)	Potassium (mg)	*Omega-3 Fat	Trans Fat	Sodium
Catsup, low sodium	1 tbsp.	16	.05/2	.02/t	.2	3.4	na	72	na	0	3
Cheese sauce, ready to serve (Nestle)	¼ cup	82	5/1.6	na	.6	.1	0	16	na	0	471
Chicken gravy, canned	¼ cup	47	3.4/.8	.9/1.5	.24	.05	0	65	na	0	343
Chicken gravy, mix, prep. w/water	¼ cup	25	1/0	.29/.35	0	.82	0	na	na	0	260
Chili sauce	1 tbsp.	16	0/0	0/0	0	2	70 mcg (BC)	36	na	0	201
Cocktail sauce (Golden Dipt)	1 tbsp.	20	0/0	na	0	na	77 mcg (BC)	na	na	0	na
Enchilada sauce	¼ cup	20	1/0	na	.4	na	130 mcg (BC)	na	na	0	na
Hollandaise sauce, dehydrated, prep. w/butter fat	1 packet	188	15.5/9	.7/4.7	0	3	37 mcg (BC)	98	na	0	1232
Horseradish	1 tbsp.	10	1/.01	.05/.01	0	1.2	0	37	na	0	47
Horseradish sauce	1 tbsp.	74	7/0	na	0	na	17 mcg (BC)	na	na	0	na
Mushroom gravy, canned	¼ cup	25	.6/.2	.6/.7	0	3.25	0	63	na	0	339
Mushroom gravy, creamy	1 cup	69	2.1/.5	.03/.27	0	1.1	0	55	na	0	1382
Mushroom gravy, mix, prep. w/o water	¼ cup	20	1/0	na	0	na	0	na	na	0	na
Mustard, brown	1 tbsp.	14	1/0	na	0	na	0	na	high	0	na

Food	Serving Size	Calories	Fat/Sat. Fat (gm)	Poly/Mono Fat (gm)	Fiber (gm)	Sugars (gm)	Carotenoids (mcg or mg)	Potassium (mg)	*Omega-3 Fat	Trans Fat	Sodium
Mustard (Grey Poupon)	1 tbsp.	19	1/.06	na	.3	na	0	na	high	0	na
Mustard, yellow	1 tsp.	3	.16/t	.03/.1	.5	.14	0	8	high	0	56
Onion gravy, mix, dry	¼ cup	77	1/.4	.03/.2	0	16.2	na	63	na	0	1005
Pesto sauce (Contadina)	¼ cup	310	30/5	na	0	na	288 mcg (BC)	na	na	0	na
Pesto sauce w/sun-dried tomato (Contadina)	¼ cup	250	24/4	na	3	na	na	na	na	0	na
Picante sauce, mild (Nestle, Ortega)	2 tbsp.	10	.07/t	.03/.01	.5	.23	127 mcg (BC)	80	na	0	252
Pork gravy mix, prep. w/water	1 serving	20	.56/.2	.02/.2	0	.83	na	16	na	0	14
Salsa, mild	2 tbsp.	7	.1/0	0/0	.5	.89	127 mcg (BC)	98	na	0	179
Salsa, black bean	2 tbsp.	10	0/0	na	1	na	na	na	na	0	na
Salsa, chunky, mild or medium (Old El Paso)	2 tbsp.	15	0/0	na	1	na	127 mcg (BC)	na	na	0	na
Salsa, green chili, mild	2 tbsp.	8	.08/0	0/0	.12	.46	27 mcg (BC)	na	na	0	172
Salsa, green jalapeno	2 tbsp.	8	2/0	0/0	0	.6	na	na	na	0	180
Stroganoff sauce	¼ cup	59	2.7/1.4	.15/.93	0	1.15	na	na	na	0	261
Sweet and sour sauce (Kikkoman)	1 tbsp.	17.5	0/0	na	0	na	0	84	na	0	na

Food	Serving Size	Calories	Fat/Sat. Fat (gm)	Poly/Mono Fat (gm)	Fiber (gm)	Sugars (gm)	Carotenoids (mcg or mg)	Potassium (mg)	*Omega-3 Fat	Trans Fat	Sodium
Sweet and sour sauce (La Choy)	1 tbsp.	29	.1/0	na	0	na	0	na	na	0	na
Tabasco sauce	¼ tsp.	.15	t/t	t/t	t	t	t	2	na	0	na
Taco sauce, canned (Old El Paso)	2 tbsp.	15	0/0	na	1	na	127 mcg (BC)	na	na	0	na
Tartar sauce (Hellman's)	1 tbsp.	70	8/1	na	0	na	8 mcg (BC)	na	na	0	na
Tartar sauce, egg-free	1 tbsp.	38	4/0	0/0	0	na	na	na	na	0	na
Tartar sauce, nonfat	1 tbsp.	10	0/0	.3/.53	0	na	8 mcg (BC)	na	na	0	na
Teriyaki sauce	1 tbsp.	16.5	t/0	na	.5	na	0	41	na	0	na
Turkey gravy, canned	¼ cup	30	1.25/.37	na	.24	5	0	109	na	0	na
Turkey gravy, nonfat (Heinz)	¼ cup	15	0/0	na	0	na	0	na	na	0	na
Turkey gravy mix, prep. w/water	¼ cup	22	1/0	na	0	na	0	na	na	0	na
White sauce, homemade	¼ cup	92	7/1.7	1.8/2.8	.1	2.73	62 mcg (BC)	93	na	0	221
Worcestershire sauce	1 tbsp.	6	0/0	na	0	1.7	11 mcg (BC)	136	na	0	167

CRACKERS

Food	Serving Size	Calories	Fat/Sat. Fat (gm)	Poly/Mono Fat (gm)	Fiber (gm)	Sugars (gm)	Carotenoids (mcg or mg)	Potassium (mg)	*Omega-3 Fat	Trans Fat	Sodium
Amaranth crackers, nonfat	8 crackers	100	0/0	na	3	na	na	na	na	0	na

Food	Serving Size	Calories	Fat/Sat. Fat (gm)	Poly/Mono Fat (gm)	Fiber (gm)	Sugars (gm)	Carotenoids (mcg or mg)	Potassium (mg)	*Omega-3 Fat	Trans Fat	Sodium
Bran crackers	7 crackers	60	3/1	na	na	na	na	na	na	0	na
Bran Thins (Nabisco)	5 crackers	120	2/0	na	2	na	0	na	na	0	na
Brown rice crackers (Eden)	4 crackers	70	4/1	na	0	na	0	na	na	0	169
Graham cracker	4 pieces	118	3/4	1/1.1	1	8.7	0	50	na	+	na
Graham snacks	7 crackers	53	.1/0	na	.6	na	0	na	na	0	na
Herb cracker, nonfat (Health Valley)	1 serving	40	0/0	na	2	na	0	na	na	0	na
Matzoh	1 matzoh	115	2/.4	na	.3	na	0	na	na	0	na
Matzoh, dietetic	1 matzoh	91	.4/0	na	.1	na	0	na	na	0	na
Matzoh, whole wheat	1 matzoh	100	.4/.07	na	3.4	na	0	na	na	0	na
Melba toast, bran	1 cracker	16	.4/.1	na	.2	na	0	na	na	0	na
Melba toast, plain	1 cracker	19.5	.16/.02	.06/.04	.3	.05	0	41	na	0	41
Melba toast rounds	4 rounds	47	.4/0	na	.8	na	0	na	na	0	na
Melba toast, wheat	1 cracker	19	.12/.08	.05/.03	.4	3.82	0	7	na	0	42
Melba toast, whole grain	1 cracker	16	.4/.1	na	.2	.2	0	na	na	0	45
Multigrain, wheat (Health Valley)	13 crackers	120	5/0	na	3	.2	0	na	na	0	na
Oat cracker (Oat Thins)	18 crackers	140	6/1	na	2*SOL	na	0	na	na	+	na
Oyster crackers	17 crackers	60	1.5/0	.17/.9	.5	.05	0	na	na	0	150
Rice cracker (Weight Watchers)	2 crackers	30	0/0	na	0	na	0	0	na	0	na

140

Food	Serving Size	Calories	Fat/Sat. Fat (gm)	Poly/Mono Fat (gm)	Fiber (gm)	Sugars (gm)	Carotenoids (mcg or mg)	Potassium (mg)	*Omega-3 Fat	Trans Fat	Sodium
Ritz cracker (Nabisco)	1 serving	79	4/.6	.28/2.9	.3	1.29	0	na	na	+	124
Ry-Crisp	2 crackers	60	0/0	na	4	na	0	na	na	0	na
Saltines (Zesta)	5 crackers	60	2/1	.18/1	0	.06	0	na	na	+	161
Saltines, multigrain (Premium)	6 crackers	85	2.3/4	.1/1.1	1	.4	0	na	na	+	na
Saltines, nonfat	6 crackers	87	.5/.07	na	1	na	0	35	na	0	na
Saltines, wheat (Zesta)	5 crackers	60	2/1	na	0	na	0	na	na	+	na
Sesame cracker (Keebler)	4 crackers	60	3/1	na	0	na	0	na	na	+	na
Sesame sticks	¼ cup	133	9/0	4.9/3	.1*SOL	13.18	t (BC)	50	high	+	8
Soda cracker	5 crackers	60	2/1	.11/1	2	.06	0	2	na	0	161
Triscuit	4 crackers	71	3.5	na	2	na	0	na	na	+	na
Triscuit, whole wheat & bran	4 crackers	70	3/.4	na	1.6	na	0	na	na	+	na
Triscuit, whole wheat, reduced fat	4 crackers	65	1.7/.3	na	2	na	0	na	na	+	na
Vegetable cracker	3 crackers	70	3/1.5	na	0	na	na	na	na	+	na
Waverly Wafers	4 crackers	80	4/.8	na	.4	na	0	na	na	+	na
Water cracker (Carr's)	2 crackers	25	1/0	na	0	na	0	na	na	0	na
Wheat cracker (Wheatsworth)	4 crackers	57	2.5/.6	na	.5	na	0	na	na	+	na

Food	Serving Size	Calories	Fat/Sat. Fat (gm)	Poly/Mono Fat (gm)	Fiber (gm)	Sugars (gm)	Carotenoids (mcg or mg)	Potassium (mg)	*Omega-3 Fat	Trans Fat	Sodium
Wheat Thins	8 crackers	70	3/1	.18/1	0	1.3	0	28	na	+	84
Wheat Thins, reduced fat	8 crackers	58	1.6/0	na	.8	na	0	na	na	+	na
DINNERS											
Amy's Kitchen (Vegetarian Meals)											
Black bean enchilada	1 meal	250	8/1	na	5*SOL	2	na	na	na	0	390
Cannelloni	1 meal	330	12/8	na	6	na	na	na	na	0	na
Cheese enchilada	1 meal	330	14/7	na	6	2	na	na	na	0	440
Chili and cornbread	1 meal	320	6/2	na	8*SOL	14	na	na	na	0	680
Country dinner	1 meal	380	12/4	na	9	14	na	na	na	0	570
Veggie loaf	1 meal	260	5/5	na	7	6	na	na	na	0	640
Healthy Choice											
Beef pot roast	1 meal	330	9/3	na	8	39	na	na	na	0	550
Beef stroganoff	1 meal	330	9/3	na	7	39	na	na	na	0	580
Beef tips portobello	1 meal	310	9/3	na	7	na	na	na	na	0	600
Blackened chicken	1 meal	320	6/2	na	5	28	na	na	na	0	600
Charbroiled beef patty	1 meal	310	9/3	na	4	36	na	na	na	0	na
Chicken broccoli Alfredo	1 meal	300	7/3	na	2	na	na	na	na	0	na
Chicken enchiladas	1 meal	270	6/3	1/2.6	6	46	na	na	na	0	563
Chicken parmigiana	1 meal	310	8/2	na	6	40	na	na	na	0	600
Chicken teriyaki	1 meal	270	6/2	.47/2.1	3	37	na	na	na	0	602

Food	Serving Size	Calories	Fat/Sat. Fat (gm)	Poly/Mono Fat (gm)	Fiber (gm)	Sugars (gm)	Carotenoids (mcg or mg)	Potassium (mg)	*Omega-3 Fat	Trans Fat	Sodium
Country breaded chicken	1 meal	380	8/2	.47/2.1	7	55	na	630	na	0	600
Country herb chicken	1 meal	280	6/3	na	6	37	na	na	na	0	600
Grilled turkey breast	1 meal	260	5/2	na	5	31	na	na	na	0	600
Herb baked fish	1 meal	360	8/2	na	5	na	na	na	high	0	na
Honey glazed chicken	1 meal	320	6/2	na	4	46	na	940	na	0	580
Lemon pepper fish	1 meal	320	7/2	na	5	46	na	na	high	0	580
Meatloaf	1 meal	330	7/3.5	na	6	36	na	na	na	0	600
Mesquite beef w/barbecue sauce	1 meal	320	9/3	2.8/3.3	5	38.3	na	na	na	0	491
Mesquite chicken BBQ	1 meal	290	5/2	.98/2	4	48.1	na	na	na	0	483
Oven roasted beef	1 meal	280	7/2.5	na	6	44	na	850	na	0	480
Roasted chicken breast	1 meal	230	6/3	na	4	33	na	na	na	0	600
Salisbury steak	1 meal	330	7/3	1.1/2.8	6	23.8	na	na	na	0	466
Sesame chicken	1 meal	330	8/2	na	5	na	na	na	high	0	na
Stuffed pasta shells	1 meal	370	6/3	na	5	40	na	na	na	0	470
Sweet and sour chicken	1 meal	360	7/2	na	3	54	na	na	na	0	580
Traditional turkey breasts	1 meal	320	5/2	na	5	50	na	na	na	0	600

Food	Serving Size	Calories	Fat/Sat. Fat (gm)	Poly/Mono Fat (gm)	Fiber (gm)	Sugars (gm)	Carotenoids (mcg or mg)	Potassium (mg)	*Omega-3 Fat	Trans Fat	Sodium
Lean Cuisine (Hearty Portions Meals)											
Beef stroganoff	1 meal	350	9/3	na	9	na	na	na	na	0	na
Cheese and spinach manicotti	1 meal	350	8/3	na	6	na	na	na	high	0	na
Chicken and barbecue	1 meal	370	6/1	na	6	na	na	na	na	0	na
Chicken fettuccini	1 meal	400	9/4.5	.5/1.5	4	6	na	510	na	0	690
Chicken florentine	1 meal	380	7/3	1.5/1.5	6	9	na	640	na	0	840
Glazed chicken	1 meal	360	8/1.5	1.5/1	2	7	na	510	na	0	690
Grilled chicken and penne pasta	1 meal	360	7/3	1/2	5	7	na	620	na	0	680
Jumbo rigatoni w/meatballs	1 meal	440	9/3.5	1/3	7	10	na	770	na	0	790
Oriental glazed chicken	1 meal	370	2/.5	.5/1	4	20	na	740	na	0	690
Roasted chicken	1 meal	330	5/1	na	4	na	na	na	na	0	na
Roasted turkey breast	1 meal	320	6/1	.5/1	6	30	na	360	na	0	690
Salisbury steak	1 meal	300	6/3	.5/2.5	8	4	na	750	na	0	650
Weight Watchers											
Barbecue Glazed Chicken	1 meal	282	4.4/1	na	na	25.9	592 mcg (BC)	na	na	0	492
Chicken Cordon Bleu	1 meal	297	9/5	na	3	na	3.8 mg	na	na	0	394
Turkey Medallions	1 meal	214	1.7/.4	.45/.43	3	34.6	na	504	na	0	392

Food	Serving Size	Calories	Fat/Sat. Fat (gm)	Poly/Mono Fat (gm)	Fiber (gm)	Sugars (gm)	Carotenoids (mcg or mg)	Potassium (mg)	*Omega-3 Fat	Trans Fat	Sodium
Macaroni and Beef in Tomato Sauce	1 meal	266	6/1.8	.98/2.3	2	na	141 mcg (BC)	na	na	0	388
DIPS											
Avocado	2 tbsp.	46	4.4/.7	na	1.4	na	104 mcg (BC)	na	na	0	na
Baba ghanoush (eggplant dip)	2 tbsp.	47	4/.5	na	.8	na	21 mcg (BC)	na	na	0	na
Bacon and horseradish	2 tbsp.	70	6/3	na	0	na	na	na	na	+	na
Bean	2 tbsp.	40	1/.5	na	2.4*SOL	na	na	51.4	na	0	.8
Black bean	2 tbsp.	20	0/0	na	1*SOL	na	60 mcg (BC)	na	na	0	na
Black bean, nonfat (Tostitos)	2 tbsp.	30	0/0	na	2*SOL	na	na	na	na	0	na
Bleu cheese	2 tbsp.	50	4/2	na	0	1.4	na	38	na	0	215
Cheddar cheese, nonfat	2 tbsp.	20	0/0	na	0	na	na	na	na	0	na
Clam (Kraft)	2 tbsp.	60	4/3	na	0	na	0	na	high	0	na
Creamy dill (Vegi-Dip)	2 tbsp.	60	4/0	na	0	na	na	na	na	0	na
Cucumber	2 tbsp.	50	4/3	na	0	na	na	na	na	0	na
Guacamole (Lucerne)	2 tbsp.	46	3/4	1/1.1	0	4	na	na	na	un	106
Hummus	2 tbsp.	51	2.6/.4	.6/1.5	1.6*SOL	.14	3.6 mcg (BC)	52	high	0	73
Nacho cheese	2 tbsp.	62	4/2	na	0	2.2	na	73	na	un	284
Onion	2 tbsp.	68	6/4	na	.3	2.5	36 mcg (BC)	57	na	un	423

Food	Serving Size	Calories	Fat/Sat. Fat (gm)	Poly/Mono Fat (gm)	Fiber (gm)	Sugars (gm)	Carotenoids (mcg or mg)	Potassium (mg)	*Omega-3 Fat	Trans Fat	Sodium
Pinto bean, nonfat (Guiltless Gourmet)	2 tbsp.	27	0/0	na	2*SOL	na	na	na	na	0	na
Shrimp	2 tbsp.	74	6/4	na	.1	na	21 mcg (BC)	43	high	un	76
Sour cream and chives	2 tbsp.	126	14/0	na	0	2.5	na	na	na	un	232
Spinach	2 tbsp.	54	4.4/1.4	na	.4	na	447 mcg (BC)	na	high	na	95.7
Vegetable (Marzetti)	2 tbsp.	176	20/0	na	0	na	na	49.8	na	un	na
EGGS											
Egg (chicken), large	1 egg	74.5	4.5/1.5	0/0	0	.23	0	67	high	0	55
White	1 large	17	0/0	0/0	0	.23	0	54	na	0	55
Yolk	1 large	59	5/1.6	.7/2	0	.1	0	19	high	0	8
Egg, cooked:											
Fried in margarine	1 large	91.5	7/2	1.2/2.9	0	.38	0	68	high	+	94
Hard-boiled, shell removed	1 large	77	5/1.6	.7/2	0	.56	0	63	high	0	62
Poached	1 large	74.5	5/1.5	.68/1.9	0	.38	0	133	high	0	147
Scrambled with milk and margarine	1 large	101	7.5/2	1.3/2.9	0	1.06	0	147	high	+	171
Egg substitutes: Cholesterol-free (Healthy Choice)	¼ cup	30	1/0	na	0	na	0	na	na	0	na
Cheese omelet Egg Beaters (Fleischmann's)	½ cup	110	5/2	na	0	na	0	na	na	0	na

Food	Serving Size	Calories	Fat/Sat. Fat (gm)	Poly/Mono Fat (gm)	Fiber (gm)	Sugars (gm)	Carotenoids (mcg or mg)	Potassium (mg)	*Omega-3 Fat	Trans Fat	Sodium
Egg Beaters (Fleischmann's)	½ cup	30	0/0	na	0	na	0	na	na	0	na
Egg Watcher's (Tofutti)	½ cup	30	0/0	na	0	na	0	256	high	0	na
Frozen Liquid Eggs (Sunny Fresh)	½ cup	130	9/3	7.5/2.9	0	3.8	0	na	na	0	239
Powdered (Tofu Scrambler-Fantastic Foods) Vegetable omelet	2½ cups	60	.5/0	na	3	na	0	na	high	0	na
Egg Beaters (Fleischmann's)	½ cup	50	0/0	na	0	na	0	na	na	0	na
Egg substitute, liquid	½ cup	105	4/.82	2/1.1	0	.8	na	414	na	0	222
Egg substitute, powdered	1 oz	126	3.7/1	.48/1.5	0	6.1	na	213	na	0	226
ENTREES											
Healthy Choice											
Beef w/barbecue sauce and rice and beans	1 entrée	250	4/5	na	2	na	na	na	na	0	na
Beef macaroni	1 entrée	220	4/2	.33/1.2	5	9.12	na	365	na	0	444
Beef teriyaki	1 entrée	330	7/2.5	na	7	17	na	na	na	0	600

Food	Serving Size	Calories	Fat/Sat. Fat (gm)	Poly/Mono Fat (gm)	Fiber (gm)	Sugars (gm)	Carotenoids (mcg or mg)	Potassium (mg)	°Omega-3 Fat	Trans Fat	Sodium
Beef tips, sirloin w/ mushroom sauce	1 entrée	270	6/2	na	4	na	na	na	na	0	na
Beef tips w/spiral pasta	1 entrée	300	7/2.5	na	4	na	na	na	na	0	na
Chicken, baked w/ mashed potatoes	1 entrée	210	4.5/1.5	na	3	na	na	na	na	0	na
Chicken breast, breaded w/mac & cheese	1 entrée	270	6/2.5	na	1	5	na	na	na	0	600
Chicken breast, grilled w/pasta	1 entrée	240	6/2.5	na	4	na	na	na	na	0	na
Chicken breast w/ vegetables	1 entrée	230	5/2	na	6	30	na	na	na	0	500
Chicken carbonara	1 entrée	310	5/2.5	na	2	32	na	na	na	0	600
Chicken, country glazed	1 entrée	250	5/2	na	3	na	na	390	na	0	600
Chicken enchilada	1 entrée	310	7/2.5	na	6	46	na	na	na	0	600
Chicken, grilled w/ mashed potatoes	1 entrée	200	4/2	na	6	25	na	na	na	0	560
Chicken, grilled Sonoma	1 entrée	230	4/1	na	3	na	na	na	na	0	na
Chicken, Mandarin	1 entrée	280	3.5/.5	na	4	na	na	na	na	0	520
Chicken ole	1 entrée	270	4/1	na	5	na	na	na	na	0	na
Chicken, oriental style	1 entrée	240	5/1.5	na	7	na	na	na	high	0	600

Food	Serving Size	Calories	Fat/Sat. Fat (gm)	Poly/Mono Fat (gm)	Fiber (gm)	Sugars (gm)	Carotenoids (mcg or mg)	Potassium (mg)	*Omega-3 Fat	Trans Fat	Sodium
Chicken and pasta, homestyle	1 entrée	270	6/2.5	na	5	38	na	na	na	0	600
Chicken piccata	1 entrée	270	5/2.5	na	2	28	na	na	na	0	600
Chicken and rice, cheesy	1 entrée	230	4/2.5	na	5	27	na	500	na	0	600
Chicken, sesame	1 entrée	240	6/2	na	4	34	na	na	high	0	580
Fettucini Alfredo	1 entrée	240	5/2.5	na	2	19	na	na	na	0	580
Fettucini Alfredo, w/ chicken	1 entrée	280	7/2.5	na	4	32	na	na	na	0	570
Lasagna	1 entrée	280	6/2	na	5	38	na	na	na	0	600
Lasagna /meat	1 entrée	360	9/3	na	7	na	na	na	na	0	na
Macaroni and cheese	1 entrée	250	6/2.5	na	3	44	na	na	na	0	600
Manicotti with three cheeses	1 entrée	300	9/3	na	5	44	na	na	na	0	600
Pizza, cheese	1 pizza	340	5/1.5	na	5	10	na	na	na	0	600
Pizza, pepperoni	1 pizza	340	5/1.5	na	6	10	na	na	na	0	600
Pizza, supreme	1 pizza	330	5/1.5	na	6	7	na	na	na	0	600
Pizza, vegetable	1 pizza	280	4/1.5	na	5	8	na	na	na	0	600
Pork, country breaded w/ cheddar bacon potatoes	1 entrée	280	6/2.5	na	4	na	na	na	na	0	na
Ravioli, cheese	1 entrée	260	5/2.5	na	4	na	na	na	na	0	na
Rigatoni w/broccoli and chicken	1 entrée	280	7/2.5	na	3	5	na	na	na	0	600

149

Food	Serving Size	Calories	Fat/Sat. Fat (gm)	Poly/Mono Fat (gm)	Fiber (gm)	Sugars (gm)	Carotenoids (mcg or mg)	Potassium (mg)	*Omega-3 Fat	Trans Fat	Sodium
Salisbury steak w/ mashed potatoes	1 entrée	210	6/2.5	na	3	6	na	na	na	0	600
Southwestern style rice and beans	1 entrée	250	3/1	na	5	na	na	na	na	0	na
Spaghetti with meatballs	1 entrée	290	8/2.5	na	7	9	na	na	na	0	600
Tuna casserole	1 entrée	240	7/2	na	4	31	na	na	high	0	600
Turkey breast, roasted	1 entrée	220	5/2	na	5	23	na	na	na	0	580
Turkey, roasted with mashed potatoes	1 entrée	200	5/2	na	4	17	na	na	na	0	600
Lean Cuisine											
Beef, Hunan beef and broccoli	1 entrée	240	3.5/1	1/2	2	6	na	530	na	0	690
Beef, oriental	1 entrée	210	3.5/1.5	.5/1	3	8	na	670	na	0	580
Beef, oven roasted	1 entrée	240	8/3.5	1/2.5	3	9	na	760	na	0	690
Beef peppercorn	1 entrée	260	7/2	1.5/2	4	8	na	890	na	0	680
Beef portobello	1 entrée	220	7/3.5	.5/1.5	2	6	na	1080	na	0	690
Beef pot roast	1 entrée	190	6/2	1/3	3	5	na	680	na	0	690
Beef tips	1 entrée	270	6/2.5	.5/2	4	11	na	1130	na	0	630
Chicken, baked	1 entrée	240	4.5/1.5	1/2	3	5	na	600	na	0	650
Chicken and bow tie pasta	1 entrée	220	4/1	1/1.5	5	6	na	700	na	0	680
Chicken carbonara	1 entrée	260	8/2	2/2	2	5	na	700	na	0	690

Food	Serving Size	Calories	Fat/Sat. Fat (gm)	Poly/Mono Fat (gm)	Fiber (gm)	Sugars (gm)	Carotenoids (mcg or mg)	Potassium (mg)	*Omega-3 Fat	Trans Fat	Sodium
Chicken chow mein	1 entrée	240	3.5/1	.5/1	3	3	na	370	na	0	620
Chicken enchilada	1 entrée	280	5/1.5	1/.5	3	7	na	370	na	0	560
Chicken, glazed	1 entrée	230	5/1	1/1.5	0	7	na	500	na	0	480
Chicken, grilled	1 entrée	250	5/1.5	2/1.5	3	4	na	540	na	0	690
Chicken, herb roasted	1 entrée	200	3.5/1	1/1	3	5	na	740	na	0	610
Chicken l'orange	1 entrée	230	1.5/.5	.5/.5	2	6	na	380	na	0	340
Chicken, Mandarin	1 entrée	240	4/1	1/1.5	2	10	na	310	na	0	610
Chicken Mediterranean	1 entrée	260	4/.5	1/1.5	4	9	na	860	na	0	690
Chicken parmesan	1 entrée	300	6/2	1/2	5	8	na	760	na	0	520
Chicken piccata	1 entrée	300	9/2.5	1/.2	2	na	na	290	na	0	670
Chicken, roasted	1 entrée	250	7/2	na	3	20	na	na	na	0	na
Chicken, sweet and sour	1 entrée	320	3/1	.5/1	1	na	na	740	na	0	690
Chicken teriyaki	1 entrée	320	3.5/1.5	.5/.5	0	9	na	820	na	0	850
Chicken w/ vegetables	1 entrée	250	5/2.5	1/1.5	3	5	na	610	na	0	630
Chicken in wine sauce	1 entrée	220	5/2.5	na	2	na	na	na	na	0	na
Fettucini Alfredo	1 entrée	280	7/3.5	1/2	2	7	na	260	na	0	670
Fish, baked, lemon pepper	1 entrée	220	6/2	0/.5	7	5	na	700	high	0	630
Lasagna, cheese	1 entrée	240	4.5/2.5	.5/1.5	5	11	na	640	na	0	690

Food	Serving Size	Calories	Fat/Sat. Fat (gm)	Poly/Mono Fat (gm)	Fiber (gm)	Sugars (gm)	Carotenoids (mcg or mg)	Potassium (mg)	*Omega-3 Fat	Trans Fat	Sodium
Lasagna w/chicken	1 entrée	280	7/3	1/2	2	7	na	660	na	0	690
Lasagna w/chicken and cheese	1 entrée	270	8/2.5	na	3	na	na	na	na	+	na
Lasagna w/meat sauce	1 entrée	300	8/4.5	.5/2	4	9	na	590	na	0	650
Lasagna, vegetable	1 entrée	260	7/3.5	1/2	4	7	na	660	na	0	670
Macaroni and cheese	1 entrée	290	7/4	.5/1.5	2	8	na	500	na	0	650
Meatloaf and whipped potatoes	1 entrée	260	7/4	.5/2.5	4	4	na	850	na	0	540
Pizza, cheese	1 pizza	340	8/4	1.5/1.5	3	8	na	250	na	0	690
Pizza, deluxe	1 pizza	330	9/3.5	1.5/1.5	3	7	na	300	na	0	590
Pizza, pepperoni	1 pizza	300	7/2.5	2/3	2	7	na	280	na	0	680
Pork, honey roasted	1 entrée	240	5/2	.5/2.5	3	8	na	370	na	0	580
Salisbury steak	1 entrée	290	9/4.5	.5/2.5	3	4	na	750	na	0	650
Santa Fe rice and beans	1 entrée	300	5/2	1/1	6*SOL	10	na	620	na	0	580
Shrimp and angel hair pasta	1 entrée	280	5/1	1.5/1.5	3	7	na	470	high	0	680
Spaghetti w/meat sauce	1 entrée	300	5/1.5	.5/1	6	9	na	470	na	0	590
Spaghetti w/ meatballs	1 entrée	270	6/2.5	.5/1.5	4	7	na	480	na	0	590
Stuffed cabbage	1 entrée	210	8/3.5	.5/1.5	5	6	na	460	na	0	620

Food	Serving Size	Calories	Fat/Sat. Fat (gm)	Poly/Mono Fat (gm)	Fiber (gm)	Sugars (gm)	Carotenoids (mcg or mg)	Potassium (mg)	*Omega-3 Fat	Trans Fat	Sodium
Swedish meatballs	1 entrée	290	7/3	1/2.5	4	5	na	580	na	0	640
Three-bean chili	1 entrée	280	8/2.5	na	8*SOL	na	na	na	na	0	na
Turkey breast, roasted	1 entrée	270	2/.5	.5/1	3	30	na	360	na	0	690
Turkey, glazed tenderloins	1 entrée	260	4.5/1	1/2	4	20	na	520	na	0	630
Lean Cuisine (Skillet Sensation Entrées)											
Beef teriyaki w/rice	1 entrée	290	4/1.5	.5/.5	6	9	na	500	na	0	540
Chicken Alfredo	1 entrée	320	7/3.5	.5/1	4	5	na	540	na	0	480
Chicken, garlic	1 entrée	340	4.5/2	na	4	na	na	na	na	0	na
Chicken, herb roasted w/potatoes	1 entrée	250	4/1	1/.5	4	7	na	430	na	0	510
Chicken, oriental	1 entrée	280	4/1	.5/.5	5	5	na	350	na	0	610
Chicken primavera	1 entrée	300	4/1	.5/.5	5	4	na	350	na	0	430
Chicken teriyaki	1 entrée	310	3.5/1.5	.5/.5	6	9	na	470	na	0	620
Chicken, three cheese	1 entrée	350	9/3.5	.5/.5	3	9	na	470	na	0	620
Turkey, roasted	1 entrée	220	2/.5	.5/.5	6	7	na	380	na	0	450
Mrs. Paul's											
Fish, Dijon light	1 entrée	200	5/2	na	0	17	na	na	high	+	na
Fish, fillet, Florentine	1 entrée	220	8/4	na	0	10	na	na	high	+	na
Fish, Mornay, light	1 entrée	230	10/4	na	0	12	na	na	high	+	na
Weight Watchers											
Beef, Sirloin and Asian Style Veg	1 entrée	230	9/4	0	3	5	na	na	na	0	750

Food	Serving Size	Calories	Fat/Sat. Fat (gm)	Poly/Mono Fat (gm)	Fiber (gm)	Sugars (gm)	Carotenoids (mcg or mg)	Potassium (mg)	*Omega-3 Fat	Trans Fat	Sodium
Chicken, Basil	1 entrée	270	6/1.5	na	2	3	na	na	na	0	700
Chicken Mirabella	1 entrée	190	1/0	4	3	4	na	na	na	0	590
Chicken, creamy parmesian	1 entrée	210	8/4.5	na	3	5	na	na	na	0	800
Chicken, Creamy Tuscan	1 entrée	180	8/3.5	na	3	5	na	na	na	0	690
Chicken, Fire-grilled w/veg.	1 entrée	280	3.5/1	na	3	12	na	380	na	0	700
Chicken, grilled in garlic herb	1 entrée	210	8/4.5	na	3	5	na	na	na	0	800
Lasagna Bolognese	1 entrée	280	4/1.5	na	4	6	na	na	na	0	540
Pasta, Fettucini Alfredo	1 entrée	270	6/3.5	na	3	7	na	na	na	0	650
Pasta, Radiatore Romano	1 entrée	280	8/3	na	4	7	na	na	na	0	510
Turkey breast, slow roasted	1 entrée	220	8/2.5	na	2	1	na	na	na	0	720
Turkey medallions w/gravy	1 entrée	200	8/1.5	na	3	3	na	na	na	0	730
Vegetarian Entrees											
Bean loaf (Natural Touch)	1 slice	160	8/1.5	na	5*SOL	na	na	na	na	0	na
Black bean vegetable enchilada (Amy's Kitchen)	1 serving	130	4/0	na	2*SOL	2	na	na	na	0	390

154

Food	Serving Size	Calories	Fat/Sat. Fat (gm)	Poly/Mono Fat (gm)	Fiber (gm)	Sugars (gm)	Carotenoids (mcg or mg)	Potassium (mg)	*Omega-3 Fat	Trans Fat	Sodium
Chik'n Vegetables											
Pot Pie, meatless (Morningstar Farms)	1 pie	350	14/3.5	na	9	na	na	na	na	0	na
Fried Chik'n w/gravy, meatless (Loma Linda)	2 pieces	160	10/1.5	na	2	na	na	na	na	0	na
Lentil rice loaf (Natural Touch)	1 slice	160	7/1	na	4	na	na	na	na	0	na
Macaroni and soy cheese (Amy's Kitchen)	1 serving	360	14/1	na	4*SOL	2	na	na	high	0	500
Salisbury steak, meatless (Amy's Kitchen)	1 entrée	420	16/5	na	9*SOL	14	na	na	na	0	570
Swiss steak, meatless (Loma Linda)	1 entrée	120	6/1	na	4*SOL	na	na	na	na	0	420
Thai stir fry w/tofu and vegetables (Amy's Kitchen)	1 entrée	270	11/7	na	2*SOL	2	na	na	high	0	na
Vegetable lasagna (Amy's Kitchen)	1 serving	280	12/4.5	na	3	5	na	na	na	0	680
Vegetable lasagna w/tofu (Amy's Kitchen)	1 serving	300	10/1	na	6	6	na	na	na	0	630

Food	Serving Size	Calories	Fat/Sat. Fat (gm)	Poly/Mono Fat (gm)	Fiber (gm)	Sugars (gm)	Carotenoids (mcg or mg)	Potassium (mg)	*Omega-3 Fat	Trans Fat	Sodium
FAST FOODS											
Breakfast Foods											
Burger King:											
Biscuit	1 biscuit	300	15/3.5	na	t	na	0	na	na	++	na
French Toast Sticks	5 sticks	390	20/4.5	na	2	11	0	na	na	++	440
Hardee's:											
Apple, Cinnamon & Raisin Biscuit	1 biscuit	250	8/2	na	na	na	0	na	na	+	na
Chicken Biscuit	1 biscuit	590	27/7	na	na	3	0	na	na	++	1680
Made from Scratch Biscuit	1 biscuit	390	21/6	na	na	3	0	na	na	+	890
Omelet Biscuit	1 biscuit	550	32/12	na	na	5	0	na	high	+	1510
Jack in the Box:											
Breakfast Jack	1 serving	310	14/5	na	1	3	0	195	na	un	715
French Toast Sticks	4 sticks	430	18/4	na	2	38	0	150	na	++	490
Sourdough Breakfast Sandwich	1 serving	450	26/8	na	2	2	0	210	na	++	875
McDonald's:											
Biscuit	1 biscuit	240	23/8	na	1	30	0	na	na	+	640
Egg McMuffin	1 serving	290	12/4.5	na	1	28	0	na	high	0	850
Lowfat Apple Bran Muffin	1 muffin	300	3/.5	na	3*SOL	na	0	na	na	un	na
Scrambled Eggs	2 eggs	160	11/3.5	na	0	1	0	na	high	0	170

156

Food	Serving Size	Calories	Fat/Sat. Fat (gm)	Poly/Mono Fat (gm)	Fiber (gm)	Sugars (gm)	Carotenoids (mcg or mg)	Potassium (mg)	*Omega-3 Fat	Trans Fat	Sodium
Spanish Omelet Bagel	1 bagel	690	38/14	na	3	59	0	na	high	un	1520
Subway:											
Ham & Egg Sandwich	1 sandwich	291	12/3	na	1	3	0	na	high	un	190
Western Egg Sandwich	1 sandwich	285	12/2.5	na	2	4	0	na	high	un	180
Burgers											
Burger King:											
WHOPPER w/o mayo	1 burger	530	22/9	na	4	8	0	na	na	+	1020
Hamburger	1 burger	320	14/6	na	2	5	0	na	na	+	550
Dairy Queen:											
DQ Homestyle Hamburger	1 burger	290	12/5	na	2	na	0	na	na	un	na
Hardee's:											
Thickburger	1 burger	270	57/22	na	na	12	0	na	na	un	1470
Jack in the Box:											
Hamburger	1 burger	250	9/3.5	na	2	6	0	115	na	un	590
Sourdough Jack	1 serving	660	47/16	na	3	7	0	435	na	+	1165
McDonald's:											
Hamburger	1 burger	280	10/4	1.3/4	2	36	0	204	na	+	502
Quarter Pounder	1 burger	430	21/8	2/10	2	38	0	385	na	+	770

Food	Serving Size	Calories	Fat/Sat. Fat (gm)	Poly/Mono Fat (gm)	Fiber (gm)	Sugars (gm)	Carotenoids (mcg or mg)	Potassium (mg)	*Omega-3 Fat	Trans Fat	Sodium
Wendy's:											
Classic Single w/Everything	1 burger	410	19/7	na	2	8	0	na	na	+	910
Desserts											
Dairy Queen:											
DQ Fudge Bar–sugar-free	1 bar	50	0/0	na	0	3	na	na	na	0	70
DQ Vanilla Orange Bar–sugar-free	1 bar	60	0/0	na	0	2	na	na	na	0	40
McDonald's:											
Fruit n' Yogurt Parfait	1 serving	380	5/2	na	2	30	0	237	na	0	85
Fruit n' Yogurt Parfait w/o granola	1 serving	280	4/2	na	t	19	0	103	na	0	55
Vanilla Reduced Fat Ice Cream Cone	1 serving	150	4.5/3	na	0	17	0	178	na	0	75
Wendy's:											
Frostie	1 small	330	8/5	na	0	42	0	150	na	0	na
Mexican Foods											
Jack in the Box:											
Monster Taco	1 taco	280	17/6	na	3	4	na	220	na	+	390
Taco	1 taco	180	10/3.5	na	2	4	na	190	na	+	270
Taco Bell:											
Burrito, Bean	1 serving	370	12/3.5	na	12*SOL	4	na	na	na	+	1200
Burrito, Chili Cheese	1 serving	330	13/5	na	4	3	na	na	na	+	1080

Food	Serving Size	Calories	Fat/Sat. Fat (gm)	Poly/Mono Fat (gm)	Fiber (gm)	Sugars (gm)	Carotenoids (mcg or mg)	Potassium (mg)	*Omega-3 Fat	Trans Fat	Sodium
Burrito, Double Supreme—Chicken	1 serving	460	17/6	na	3	na	na	na	na	+	na
Burrito, Fiesta—Chicken	1 serving	370	12/3.5	na	3	3	na	na	na	+	1080
Burrito—7-Layer	1 serving	520	22/7	na	13*SOL	6	na	na	na	+	1350
Burrito, Supreme—Chicken	1 serving	410	16/6	na	8	5	na	na	na	+	1270
Chalupa Baja—Chicken	1 serving	400	24/5	na	2	4	na	na	na	+	690
Chalupa Nacho Cheese—Chicken	1 serving	350	19/4.5	na	2	4	na	na	na	+	670
Chalupa Santa Fe—Chicken	1 serving	420	26/6	na	2	na	na	na	na	+	na
Chalupa Supreme—Chicken	1 serving	360	20/7	na	2	4	na	na	na	+	530
Enchirito, Chicken	1 serving	350	16/8	na	7	na	na	na	na	+	na
Gordita Baja—Chicken	1 serving	340	18/4	na	3	7	na	na	na	+	690
Gordita Nacho Cheese—Chicken	1 serving	290	13/2.5	na	3	7	na	na	na	un	670
Gordita Santa Fe—Chicken	1 serving	370	20/4	na	3	na	na	na	na	un	na
Gordita Supreme—Chicken	1 serving	300	13/5	na	3	na	na	na	na	un	530
Taco	1 taco	210	12/4	na	3	1	na	na	na	un	350

Food	Serving Size	Calories	Fat/Sat. Fat (gm)	Poly/Mono Fat (gm)	Fiber (gm)	Sugars (gm)	Carotenoids (mcg or mg)	Potassium (mg)	*Omega-3 Fat	Trans Fat	Sodium
Taco, Double Decker	1 taco	380	17/5	na	9	na	na	na	na	un	na
Taco, Double Decker Supreme	1 taco	420	21/8	na	10	na	na	na	na	un	na
Taco, Soft–Chicken	1 taco	190	7/2.5	na	2	na	na	na	na	un	na
Taco Supreme	1 taco	260	16/6	na	4	9	na	na	na	un	360
Tostada	1 serving	250	12/4.5	na	11	na	na	na	na	un	na
Pasta											
Fazoli's:											
Baked Ravioli w/ Meat Sauce	1 serving	790	29/15	na	6	8	na	na	na	0	800
Baked Rigatoni	1 serving	470	18/8	na	4	na	na	na	na	0	na
Baked Ziti–Regular	1 serving	750	26/11	na	6	na	na	na	na	0	na
Broccoli Fettuccine Alfredo	1 serving	560	15/4	na	6	5	na	na	na	0	190
Broccoli Lasagna	1 serving	420	18/5	na	5	12	na	na	na	0	1860
Lasagna	1 serving	440	19/6	na	4	13	na	na	na	0	1940
Manicotti w/Tomato Sauce	1 serving	290	15/8	na	2	na	na	na	na	0	na
Spaghetti w/Tomato Sauce--regular	1 serving	620	8/1	na	7	12	na	na	na	0	140
Pizza Hut:											
Cavatini Pasta	1 serving	480	14/6	na	9	.3	na	na	na	0	950
Spaghetti w/ Marinara	1 serving	490	6/1	na	8	.7	na	na	na	0	1050

Food	Serving Size	Calories	Fat/Sat. Fat (gm)	Poly/Mono Fat (gm)	Fiber (gm)	Sugars (gm)	Carotenoids (mcg or mg)	Potassium (mg)	*Omega-3 Fat	Trans Fat	Sodium
Spaghetti w/ Meatballs	1 serving	850	24/10	na	10	.7	na	na	na	0	1610
Pizza											
Fazoli's:											
Cheese Pizza	1 slice	460	15/8	na	2	6	na	na	na	0	970
Combination Pizza	1 slice	570	25/12	na	3	7	na	na	na	0	1360
Pizza Hut:											
Cheese	1 slice	240	10/5	na	2	na	0	na	na	un	na
Chicken Supreme	1 slice	230	7/3.5	na	2	na	0	na	na	un	na
Veggie Lover's	1 slice	220	8/3	na	2	na	na	na	na	un	na
Poultry (including chicken sandwiches)											
Arby's:											
Chicken Breast Fillet Sandwich	1 serving	540	30/5	na	2	7	0	na	na	+	1220
Chicken Cordon Bleu Sandwich	1 serving	630	35/8	na	2	8	0	na	na	+	1880
Grilled Chicken Deluxe Sandwich	1 serving	450	22/4	na	2	9	0	na	na	+	920
Light Grilled Chicken Sandwich	1 serving	280	5/1.5	na	3	na	0	na	na	+	na
Light Roast Chicken Deluxe Sandwich	1 serving	260	5/.5	na	3	na	0	na	na	+	na
Burger King:											
Fish Fillet w/Cheese	1 serving	520	30/8	na	3	4	0	na	high	+	840

161

Food	Serving Size	Calories	Fat/Sat. Fat (gm)	Poly/Mono Fat (gm)	Fiber (gm)	Sugars (gm)	Carotenoids (mcg or mg)	Potassium (mg)	*Omega-3 Fat	Trans Fat	Sodium
Chicken Sandwich w/o mayo	1 serving	460	17/5	na	3	5	0	na	na	+	1270
Dairy Queen:											
Breaded Chicken Sandwich	1 serving	510	27/4	na	2	9	0	na	na	un	1070
Grilled Chicken Sandwich	1 serving	310	10/2.5	na	3	na	0	na	na	un	na
Hardee's:											
Breast	1 piece	370	15/4	na	na	0	0	na	na	un	1190
Spicey Chicken Sandwich	1 serving	470	26/5	na	na	6	0	na	na	un	1220
Low Carb Charbroiled Chicken Club	1 serving	420	24/7	na	na	8	0	na	na	un	1230
Leg	1 piece	170	7/2	na	na	0	0	na	na	un	570
Jack in the Box:											
Chicken Breast Pieces	5 pieces	360	17/3	na	1	1	0	545	na	+	1470
Chicken Fajita Pita	1 serving	330	11/4.5	na	3	4	0	500	na	+	1080
Chicken Sandwich	1 serving	410	21/4.5	na	2	3	0	245	na	+	730
Chicken Supreme	1 serving	710	39/11	na	4	na	0	na	na	+	na
Chicken Teriyaki Bowl	1 serving	550	3/5	na	3	na	0	na	na	+	na
Grilled Chicken Fillet	1 serving	430	22/6	na	2	na	0	na	na	+	na

Food	Serving Size	Calories	Fat/Sat. Fat (gm)	Poly/Mono Fat (gm)	Fiber (gm)	Sugars (gm)	Carotenoids (mcg or mg)	Potassium (mg)	*Omega-3 Fat	Trans Fat	Sodium
Jack's Spicy Chicken	1 serving	580	31/6	na	3	7	0	460	na	+	1090
Fazoli's:											
Chicken Caesar Club Panini	1 serving	660	35/11	na	3	1	na	na	na	0	1670
Chicken Pesto Panini	1 serving	510	20/6	na	3	1	na	na	na	0	1350
Smoked Turkey Panini	1 serving	710	38/12	na	3	3	na	na	na	0	2110
Kentucky Fried Chicken:											
Hot & Spicy Chicken–Breast	1 piece	505	29/8	na	1	0	0	na	na	+	1450
Original Recipe Chicken–Breast	1 piece	400	24/6	na	1	0	0	na	na	+	1150
Original Recipe Sandwich w/o sauce	1 serving	360	13/3.5	na	t	0	0	na	na	+	890
Tender Roast Chicken Sandwich w/o sauce	1 serving	270	5/1.5	na	1	2	0	na	na	+	1510
Long John Silvers:											
Chicken Sandwich	1 sandwich	340	14/3.5	na	na	4	0	na	na	un	810
McDonald's:											
Chicken McGrill w/o mayo	1 sandwich	340	7/1.5	na	2	7	0	505	na	0	1240
Chicken McNuggets	4 pieces	170	10/2	na	0	0	0	161	na	+	450

163

Food	Serving Size	Calories	Fat/Sat. Fat (gm)	Poly/Mono Fat (gm)	Fiber (gm)	Sugars (gm)	Carotenoids (mcg or mg)	Potassium (mg)	*Omega-3 Fat	Trans Fat	Sodium
Wendy's:											
Chicken Breast Fillet Sandwich	1 sandwich	430	16/3	na	2	8	0	na	na	+	1320
Chicken Club Sandwich	1 sandwich	470	20/4.5	na	2	na	0	na	na	+	na
Homestyle Chicken Strips	3 pieces	410	18/3.5	na	0	0	0	na	na	+	1470
Grilled Chicken Sandwich	1 sandwich	300	7/1.5	na	2	11	0	na	na	+	1100
Spicy Chicken Sandwich	1 sandwich	410	14/2.5	na	2	8	0	na	na	+	1480
**Salads											
Arby's:											
Caesar Salad	1 serving	90	4/2.5	na	3	na	na	na	na	0	na
Caesar Side Salad	1 serving	45	2/1	na	2	na	na	na	na	0	na
Garden Salad	1 serving	70	1/0	na	6	2	na	na	na	0	na
Grilled Chicken Caesar Salad	1 serving	230	8/3.5	na	3	na	na	na	na	+	na
Asian Sesame Salad	1 serving	140	10/1	na	3	11	na	na	high	0	360
Roast Chicken Salad	1 serving	160	2.5/0	na	6	na	na	na	na	0	na
Side Salad	1 serving	25	0/0	na	2	3	na	na	na	0	25

*Dressing not included except where noted

164

Food	Serving Size	Calories	Fat/Sat. Fat (gm)	Poly/Mono Fat (gm)	Fiber (gm)	Sugars (gm)	Carotenoids (mcg or mg)	Potassium (mg)	*Omega-3 Fat	Trans Fat	Sodium
Martha's Vineyard Salad	1 serving	250	8/4.5	na	4	23	na	na	na	0	490
Jack in the Box:											
Side Salad	1 serving	50	3/1.5	na	2	3	na	210	na	0	290
Fazoli's:											
Chicken & Pasta Caesar Salad	1 serving	370	13/3	na	3	7	na	na	na	0	920
Garden Salad	1 serving	30	0/0	na	2	4	na	na	na	0	20
Italian Chef Salad	1 serving	260	21/9	na	3	3	na	na	na	0	1450
Pasta Salad w/ dressing	1 serving	600	26/7	na	5	13	na	na	na	0	2010
Side Pasta Salad w/dressing	1 serving	240	10/3	na	2	4	na	na	na	0	580
McDonald's:											
Grilled Chicken Bacon Ranch Salad	1 serving	250	10/4.5	na	3	3	na	763	na	na	930
California Cobb Salad w/o chicken	1 serving	150	9/4.5	na	2	3	na	439	na	na	410
Grilled Chicken Caesar Salad	1 serving	100	2.5/1.5	na	2	3	na	783	na	0	820
Quizno's:											
Tuscan Chicken Salad	1 serving	326	6.3/1	na	4	na	na	na	na	un	na

165

Food	Serving Size	Calories	Fat/Sat. Fat (gm)	Poly/Mono Fat (gm)	Fiber (gm)	Sugars (gm)	Carotenoids (mcg or mg)	Potassium (mg)	*Omega-3 Fat	Trans Fat	Sodium
Subway (Lower fat):											
Ham	1 serving	112	3/1	na	3	8	na	na	na	0	1270
Roast Beef	1 serving	114	3/.5	na	3	8	na	na	na	0	910
Roasted Chicken Breast	1 serving	137	3/.5	na	3	9	na	na	na	0	1010
Subway Club	1 serving	145	3.5/1	na	3	na	na	na	na	0	na
Tuna w/light mayo	1 serving	238	16/4	na	3	na	na	na	high	0	na
Turkey Breast	1 serving	105	2/.5	na	3	7	na	na	na	0	1010
Turkey Breast & Ham	1 serving	117	3/.5	na	3	8	na	na	na	0	1220
Veggie Delite	1 serving	50	1/0	na	3	7	na	na	na	0	510
Taco Bell:											
Taco Salad w/Salsa	1 serving	850	52/14	n	16	10	na	na	na	+	1780
Taco Salad w/Salsa, no shell	1 serving	400	22/10	na	15	9	na	na	na	0	1520
Wendy's:											
Caesar Side Salad	1 serving	110	5/2.5	na	1	1	na	na	na	0	190
Spring Mix Salad	1 serving	180	11/6	na	4	5	na	na	na	0	230
Mandarin Chicken Salad	1 serving	190	3/1	na	4	11	na	na	na	un	740
Side Salad	1 serving	60	3/.5	na	2	4	na	na	na	0	21
Taco Salad	1 serving	380	19/10	na	8	8	na	na	na	un	1090

Food	Serving Size	Calories	Fat/Sat. Fat (gm)	Poly/Mono Fat (gm)	Fiber (gm)	Sugars (gm)	Carotenoids (mcg or mg)	Potassium (mg)	*Omega-3 Fat	Trans Fat	Sodium
Sandwiches (Other)											
Arby's:											
Arby-Q	1 serving	360	14/4	na	2	20	0	na	na	+	1210
Regular Roast Beef	1 serving	350	16/6	na	2	5	0	na	na	+	950
Roast Chicken Caesar	1 serving	820	38/9	na	5	na	0	na	na	+	na
Roast Turkey & Swiss	1 serving	760	33/6	na	5	5	0	na	na	+	1790
Hardee's:											
Big Roast Beef	1 serving	410	24/9	na	na	3	0	na	na	un	1290
Regular Roast Beef	1 serving	310	16/6	na	na	2	0	na	na	un	860
Seafood (including fish sandwiches)											
Hardee's:											
Fisherman's Fillet	1 sandwich	530	28/7	na	na	na	0	na	high	un	na
Long John Silvers:											
Breaded Clams	1 order	250	14/3.5	na	na	5	0	na	high	un	1100
Country Style Breaded Fish	1 piece	200	13/4	na	na	0	0	na	high	un	700
Crabcake	1 crabcake	150	9/2	na	na	0	0	na	high	un	390
Flatbread Sandwich (Fish)	1 sandwich	740	48/9	na	na	na	0	na	high	un	na
Fish Sandwich	1 sandwich	430	20/5	na	na	4	0	na	high	un	1120
Lemon Crumb Fish	2 pieces	240	12/4	na	na	na	0	na	high	un	na

Food	Serving Size	Calories	Fat/Sat. Fat (gm)	Poly/Mono Fat (gm)	Fiber (gm)	Sugars (gm)	Carotenoids (mcg or mg)	Potassium (mg)	*Omega-3 Fat	Trans Fat	Sodium
Lemon Crumb Fish Meal	1 meal	730	29/6	na	na	na	na	na	high	un	na
Ultimate Fish Sandwich	1 sandwich	480	25/10	na	na	4	na	na	high	un	1310
McDonald's:											
Sides											
Arby's:											
Filet-O-Fish	1 sandwich	470	26/5	na	1	5	0	na	high	+	245
Broccoli 'N Cheddar Baked Potato	1 potato	540	24/12	na	7	6	na	na	high	un	780
Deluxe Baked Potato	1 potato	650	34/20	na	6	5	na	na	na	0	750
Hardee's:											
Cole Slaw	1 serving	240	20/3	na	na	na	na	na	na	0	na
Mashed Potatoes	1 small serving	70	t/t	na	na	1	na	na	na	0	410
Kentucky Fried Chicken:											
BBQ Baked Beans	5½ oz.	190	3/1	na	6*SOL	22	na	na	na	0	720
Cole Slaw	5 oz	232	13.5/2	na	3	13	na	na	na	0	300
Corn on the Cob	5.7 oz.	150	1.5/0	na	2	10	na	na	na	0	10
Green Beans	4.7 oz.	45	1.5	na	.5*SOL	2	na	na	na	0	460
Mashed Potatoes w/ gravy	4.8 oz.	120	6/1	na	2	1	na	na	na	un	380
Mean Greens	5.4 oz.	70	3/1	na	5	na	na	na	na	0	na

168

Food	Serving Size	Calories	Fat/Sat. Fat (gm)	Poly/Mono Fat (gm)	Fiber (gm)	Sugars (gm)	Carotenoids (mcg or mg)	Potassium (mg)	*Omega-3 Fat	Trans Fat	Sodium
Long John Silvers:											
Cole Slaw	4 oz.	170	70/7	na	na	10	na	na	na	0	340
Corn Cobbette	1 cobbette	80	.5/0	na	na	6	na	na	na	0	0
Rice	4 oz.	180	4/5	na	na	1	na	na	na	0	540
Taco Bell:											
Mexican Rice	4½ oz.	190	9/3.5	na	t*SOL	1	na	na	na	0	740
Pinto Beans 'n Cheese	4½ oz.	180	8/4	na	10*SOL	1	na	na	na	0	700
Wendy's:											
Baked Potato, Broccoli & Cheese	10 oz.	470	14/3	na	9	6	na	na	high	0	540
Baked Potato, Plain	10 oz.	310	0/0	na	6	3	na	na	na	0	25
Soup/Chili											
Fazoli's:											
Minestrone Soup	1 serving	120	1/0	na	8	8	na	na	na	0	910
Long John Silvers:											
Clam Chowder	1 bowl	520	24/10	na	na	8	na	high	na	un	810
Subway:											
Black Bean	1 cup	180	4.5/2	na	15*SOL	na	na	na	na	un	na
Brown and Wild Rice w/Chicken	1 cup	190	11/4.5	na	2	3	na	na	na	un	990
Chicken and Dumpling	1 cup	130	4.5/2.5	na	1	2	na	na	na	un	1030

Food	Serving Size	Calories	Fat/Sat. Fat (gm)	Poly/Mono Fat (gm)	Fiber (gm)	Sugars (gm)	Carotenoids (mcg or mg)	Potassium (mg)	*Omega-3 Fat	Trans Fat	Sodium
Cream of Potato w/Bacon	1 cup	210	12/4	na	4	3	na	na	na	un	840
Golden Broccoli Cheese	1 cup	180	12/4	na	9	3	na	high	na	un	1120
Minestrone	1 cup	70	1/0	na	0	1	na	na	na	un	1180
New England Clam Chowder	1 cup	140	4.5/1	na	1	1	na	high	na	un	990
Potato Cheese Chowder	1 cup	210	10/7	na	2	na	na	na	na	un	na
Roasted Chicken Noodle	1 cup	90	4/1	na	1	1	na	na	na	un	940
Tomato Bisque	1 cup	90	2.5/.5	na	3	na	na	na	na	un	na
Vegetable Beef	1 cup	90	1.5/.5	na	2	3	na	na	na	un	1050
Wendy's:											
Chili, small	8 oz.	227	7/2.5	na	5*SOL	5	na	na	na	un	870
Chili, large	12 oz.	340	10/3.5	na	7*SOL	7	na	na	na	un	1310
Subs											
Arby's:											
French Dip	1 sub	440	18/8	na	2	5	0	na	na	+	2040
Roast Beef	1 sub	760	48/16	na	3	2	0	na	na	+	950
Turkey	1 sub	630	37/9	na	2	na	0	na	na	+	na
Fazoli's:											
Submarino Original	1 sub	1160	55/17	na	8	8	na	na	na	0	3320
Submarino Turkey	1 sub	990	34/10	na	7	8	0	na	na	0	2500

Food	Serving Size	Calories	Fat/Sat. Fat (gm)	Poly/Mono Fat (gm)	Fiber (gm)	Sugars (gm)	Carotenoids (mcg or mg)	Potassium (mg)	*Omega-3 Fat	Trans Fat	Sodium
Submarino Veggie	1 sub	1150	55/13	na	8	na	na	na	na	0	na
Quizno's:											
Honey Bourbon Sub	1 small sub	329	6/1	na	3	45	0	na	na	0	1494
Turkey Lite Sub	1 small sub	334	6/1	na	3	52	0	na	na	0	1909
Veggie Lite	1 small sub	300	6/1	na	5	na	na	na	na	0	na
Subway (Lowfat):											
Ham	6" sub	261	4.5/1.5	na	3	8	0	na	na	0	1270
Honey Mustard Turkey w/ Cucumber	6" sub	275	3.5/1	na	2	na	0	na	na	0	na
Roast Beef	6" sub	264	4.5/1	na	3	8	0	na	na	0	910
Roasted Chicken Breast	6" sub	311	6/1.5	na	3	9	0	na	na	0	1010
Subway Club	6" sub	294	5/1.5	na	3	na	0	na	na	0	na
Turkey Breast	6" sub	254	3.5/1	na	3	7	0	na	na	0	1010
Turkey Breast & Ham	6" sub	267	4.5/1	na	3	8	0	na	na	0	1220
Veggie Delite	6" sub	200	2.5/.5	na	3	7	na	na	na	0	510
FATS & OILS											
Beef tallow	1 tbsp.	115	13/6	.51/5.3	0	0	0	0	na	0	0
Butter:											
Stick	1 pat	36	4/2.5	.15/1	0	0	24 mcg (BC)	1	na	0	29
Whipped, stick	1 pat	27	3/2	.1/.8	0	0	19 mcg (BC)	1	na	0	31

171

Food	Serving Size	Calories	Fat/Sat. Fat (gm)	Poly/Mono Fat (gm)	Fiber (gm)	Sugars (gm)	Carotenoids (mcg or mg)	Potassium (mg)	*Omega-3 Fat	Trans Fat	Sodium
Whipped, tub	1 tbsp.	67	7.6/4.7	na	0	0	47 mcg (BC)	2	na	0	78
Butter, light:											
Stick	1 pat	25	2.8/1.7	.1/.79	0	0	58 mcg (BC)	4	na	0	23
Whipped, tub	1 tbsp.	47	5/3.3	na	0	0	110 mcg (BC)	na	na	0	na
Butter-margarine blend:											
Stick	1 pat	36	4/1.7	.9/1.6	0	0	33 mcg (BC)	2	na	‡‡	na
Tub	1 tbsp.	102	11.5/4	na	0	0	117 mcg (BC)	na	na	‡‡	na
Butter replacement, powdered:											
Molly McButter	1 tbsp.	23	.1/0	na	0	0	0	na	na	0	na
Lard	1 tbsp.	115	13/5	1.4/5.8	0	0	0	0	na	0	0
Margarine:											
Corn, hard	1 pat	34	3.7/.7	.83/2.1	0	0	na	2	na	‡‡	44
Corn & soybean	1 pat	34	3.7/.7	1.2/1.7	0	0	na	1	na	‡‡	0
Liquid, soybean	1 tbsp.	102	11/2	5/4	0	0	na	13	na	+	111
Lower calorie	1 tbsp.	50	8/5.6	2.6/.85	0	0	na	2	na	+	80
Nonfat	1 tbsp.	5	.2/0	.26/1	0	0	0	8	na	0	125
Soybean, hard	1 pat	34	3.8/.6	1.2/1.7	0	0	na	2	na	‡‡	44
Soybean, soft	1 tbsp.	100	11/2.4	.3/1.8	0	0	na	1	na	+	48
Spread, extra light (Weight Watchers)	1 tbsp.	50	6/1	na	0	0	na	na	na	+	na
Stick, regular	1 tbsp	99	11/2	3.2/5.2	0	0	41 mcg (BC)	3	na	‡‡	92
Super light (Smart Beat)	1 tbsp.	20	2/0	.66/.8	0	0	na	1	na	0	46
Tub	1 tbsp.	102	11/2	3.9/5.1	0	0	117 mcg (BC)	5	na	‡‡	153

Food	Serving Size	Calories	Fat/Sat. Fat (gm)	Poly/Mono Fat (gm)	Fiber (gm)	Sugars (gm)	Carotenoids (mcg or mg)	Potassium (mg)	*Omega-3 Fat	Trans Fat	Sodium
Whipped, tub	1 tbsp.	67	7.6/1.2	na	0	0	77 mcg (BC)	na	na	+	na
Margarine-like spread:											
40% fat	1 tbsp.	50	5.6/.9	.59/.52	0	0	na	1	na	++	35
60% fat	1 tsp.	26	2.9/.58	.34/.19	0	0	na	na	na	++	48
Shortening (Crisco)	1 tbsp.	110	12/3	na	0	0	0	na	na	0	na
Vegetable oil spreads:											
I Can't Believe It's Not Butter	1 tbsp.	90	10/2	na	0	0	118 mcg	na	na	++	na
Promise	1 tbsp.	35	4/0	na	0	0	118 mcg	na	na	+	na
Squeezable	1 tbsp.	80	9/1.5	na	0	0	na	na	na	+	na
Oils:											
Canola	1 tbsp.	122	13.6/1	4.1/8.2	0	0	na	na	high	0	na
Corn	1 tbsp.	120	14/2	7.4/3.7	0	0	na	na	high	0	na
**Flax seed	1 tbsp.	120	13.6/1.3	9/2.7	0	0	0	na	high	0	na
Grapeseed	1 tbsp.	120	13.6/1.3	9.5/2.2	0	0	na	na	high	0	na
Olive	1 tbsp.	120	14/0	1.3/10	0	0	na	na	high	0	na
Peanut	1 tbsp.	122	13.6/2.5	4.3/6.2	0	0	na	na	high	0	na
Popcorn oil	1 tbsp.	120	14/2	4.3/6.2	0	0	na	na	high	0	na
Safflower, linoleic over 70%	1 tbsp.	120	13.6/.8	10/1.9	0	0	na	na	high	0	na
Soybean	1 tbsp.	122	13.6/2	7.9/3.2	0	0	na	na	high	0	na
Sunflower	1 tbsp.	120	13.6/1.4	4.9/6.3	0	0	na	na	high	0	na

**Available in high-lignan formulations

173

Food	Serving Size	Calories	Fat/Sat. Fat (gm)	Poly/Mono Fat (gm)	Fiber (gm)	Sugars (gm)	Carotenoids (mcg or mg)	Potassium (mg)	*Omega-3 Fat	Trans Fat	Sodium
Vegetable	1 tbsp.	122	13.6/2	na	0	0	na	na	high	0	na
Wheat germ	1 tbsp.	120	13.6/2.5	8.4/2	0	0	na	na	high	0	na
FISH & SHELLFISH											
Anchovy, canned in olive oil	6 fillets	25	1.5/0	.5/.75	0	0	0	109	high	0	734
Bass, baked or broiled	1 fillet	90	3/.6	.84/1.1	0	0	0	283	high	0	56
Bluefish	3 oz.	135	4.6/1	.9/1.5	0	0	0	316	high	0	51
Catfish, breaded, fried	3 oz.	195	11/3	2.8/1	0	6.8	0	289	high	un	238
Catfish, cooked	3 oz.	129	7/1.5	.54/.93	0	0	0	356	high	0	43
Clams, canned	¼ cup	50	1.5/.5	na	0	0	0	na	high	0	na
Clams, breaded, fried	½ cup	301	17.6/4.4	4.5/7.6	0	25.8	0	177	high	un	556
Cod, Atlantic, cooked	3 oz.	89	.7/.14	.25/.1	0	0	0	207	high	un	66
Crab cake	1 cake	93	4.5/.9	1.4/1.7	0	0	0	194	high	un	198
Crab, Alaska King, cooked	3 oz.	82	1.3/.1	.46/16	0	.29	0	223	high	0	911
Crab, blue, canned	1 can (6.5 oz.)	124	1.5/.3	.55/.27	0	0	0	468	high	0	416
Crab, imitation	½ cup	80	1/0	na	0	0	0	na	high	0	na
Fish, packaged: Breaded, frozen (Van de Kamp's)	2 pieces	280	18/3	na	0	na	0	na	high	+	na

174

Food	Serving Size	Calories	Fat/Sat. Fat (gm)	Poly/Mono Fat (gm)	Fiber (gm)	Sugars (gm)	Carotenoids (mcg or mg)	Potassium (mg)	*Omega-3 Fat	Trans Fat	Sodium
Sticks, breaded, frozen (Van de Kamp's)	4 pieces	200	12/2	na	0	na	0	na	.	+	na
Flounder, frozen, cooked	3 oz.	88	1.7/0	.55/.24	0	0	0	292	high	0	84
Grouper, cooked	3 oz.	100	1/.25	.34/.22	0	0	0	404	high	0	45
Haddock, cooked	3 oz.	95	.8/.14	.3/.15	0	0	0	399	high	0	87
Halibut, cooked	3 oz.	119	2.5/.35	.8/.82	0	0	0	490	high	0	59
Herring, pickled	1 cup	367	25/3	2.3/16.7	0	0	0	97	high	0	1218
Lobster meat	1 cup	142	1/.5	.13/.23	0	0	0	510	high	0	551
Mackerel, cooked	3 oz.	223	15/3.5	3.6/5.9	0	0	0	341	high	0	71
Mahi Mahi (Peter Pan Seafoods)	3.5 oz fillets	85	.7/0	na	0	0	0	na	high	un	na
Ocean perch, cooked	3 oz.	103	1.8/.3	.46/.68	0	0	0	298	high	0	82
Orange roughy	3 oz.	76	.8/.02	.01/.5	0	na	0	327	high	0	69
Oysters:											
Breaded, fried	6 medium	173	11/3	4.6/6.9	na	39.8	0	182	high	+	677
Canned, smoked, cottonseed oil (Reese)	1 can	170	9/4	na	0	na	0	na	high	0	na
Raw	6 medium	50	1.3/.4	.5/.13	0	4.65	0	104	high	0	150
Steamed	6 medium	47	1.3/.4	na	0	na	0	na	high	0	na
Pollock, cooked	1 fillet	68	.7/.1	.93/.22	0	0	0	689	high	0	166

Food	Serving Size	Calories	Fat/Sat. Fat (gm)	Poly/Mono Fat (gm)	Fiber (gm)	Sugars (gm)	Carotenoids (mcg or mg)	Potassium (mg)	*Omega-3 Fat	Trans Fat	Sodium
Salmon:											
Cooked	3 oz.	175	11/2	3.8/3.8	0	0	31	326	high	0	52
Pink, Atlantic, canned, w/o salt	3.5 oz.	140	6/2	2/1.8	0	0	0	323	high	0	74
Smoked	3 oz.	120	6/2	na	0	na	0	na	high	0	na
Sardines:											
Canned in mustard sauce (Underwood)	3.75 oz.	220	16/0	na	0	na	0	na	high	0	na
Canned in oil	3 oz.	240	20/0	4.7/3.6	0	0	0	365	high	0	465
Canned in tomato sauce (Underwood)	3.75 oz.	220	16/0	1.9/4.3	0	.38	t	303	high	0	368
Canned in water	3 oz.	230	18/0	na	0	na	0	na	high	0	na
Scallops:											
Baked or broiled	1 cup	253	7.5/1.3	na	0	na	0	na	high	0	na
Floured or breaded, fried	6 pieces	386	19/5	6/12.5	.4	38.5	0	294	high	+	919
Shrimp:											
Breaded, fried	4 large	73	4/6	1.5/1.1	.11	3.44	0	68	high	+	103
Butterfly, frozen (Gorton's)	4 oz.	160	1/0	na	0	na	0	na	high	0	na
Canned	10 shrimp	38	.6/.1	.2/.08	0	na	0	60	high	0	48
Steamed	4 large	22	.2/.06	.09/.04	0	na	0	40	high	0	49
Snapper, cooked	1 fillet	218	3/6	1.5/na	0	na	0	887	high	0	97

176

Food	Serving Size	Calories	Fat/Sat. Fat (gm)	Poly/Mono Fat (gm)	Fiber (gm)	Sugars (gm)	Carotenoids (mcg or mg)	Potassium (mg)	*Omega-3 Fat	Trans Fat	Sodium
Sole, frozen, cooked (Gorton's)	5 oz.	110	1/0	na	0	na	0	na	high	0	na
Squid, fried	3 oz.	149	6/1.5	1.8/2.3	0	6.6	0	237	high	0	260
Surimi	3 oz.	84	.8/.15	.37/.13	0	0	0	95	high	0	122
Swordfish, baked	1 piece	164	5.5/1.5	1.2/2.1	0	0	0	391	high	0	122
Trout	1 fillet	118	5/1	1.2/2.6	0	0	0	287	high	0	42
Tuna:											
Canned in oil, light	3 oz.	167	9/1.5	2.4/2.5	0	0	0	176	high	0	301
Canned in water, light	3 oz.	106	2/0	.29/.13	0	0	0	201	high	0	287
Canned in water, white	3 oz.	123	2/0	.94/.67	0	0	0	na	high	0	na
Steak (SeaPak)	6 oz.	180	2/0	na	0	na	0	201	high	0	320

FLOUR & GRAINS

Flours

Food	Serving Size	Calories	Fat/Sat. Fat (gm)	Poly/Mono Fat (gm)	Fiber (gm)	Sugars (gm)	Carotenoids (mcg or mg)	Potassium (mg)	*Omega-3 Fat	Trans Fat	Sodium
Barley flour	1 cup	511	2.3/5	1.1/.3	4.4*SOL	1.2	na	457	na	0	6
Blue corn flour	1 cup	520	6/0	na	12	na	na	na	na	0	na
Brown rice flour	1 cup	574	4.4/.9	1.6/1.6	7	120.8	0	457	na	0	13
Buckwheat flour	1 cup	402	3.7/.8	1.1/1.1	12	3.1	na	692	na	0	13
Carob flour	1 cup	229	.7/.09	.22/.2	41	50	6 mcg (BC)	852	na	0	36
Chick pea flour	1 cup	339	6/6	2.7/1.4	10*SOL	10	na	778	na	0	59
Corn flour, masa	1 cup	416	4/6	2/1.1	11	.73	na	340	na	0	6
Corn flour, white, whole grain	1 cup	422	4.6/6	2/1.2	11	.75	na	369	na	0	6

177

Food	Serving Size	Calories	Fat/Sat. Fat (gm)	Poly/Mono Fat (gm)	Fiber (gm)	Sugars (gm)	Carotenoids (mcg or mg)	Potassium (mg)	*Omega-3 Fat	Trans Fat	Sodium
Corn flour, yellow, whole grain	1 cup	422	4.5/.6	2/1.2	16	.75	na	369	na	0	6
Graham flour	1 cup	360	20/0	na	16	na	na	na	na	0	na
Kamut flour	1 cup	440	0/0	na	16	na	na	na	na	0	na
Oat flour	1 cup	400	8/0	na	t	na	na	na	na	0	na
Oat bran flour	½ cup	76	2.2/.4	.9/.7	.67*SOL	20	na	200	na	0	170
Peanut flour, defatted	1 cup	196	.3/.03	.08/.13	9.5	4.9	na	774	high	0	108
Peanut flour, low fat	1 cup	257	13/2	4.1/6.5	9.5	18.76	na	815	high	0	1
Potato flour	1 cup	571	.5/.15	.24/.01	9	5.6	na	1602	na	0	88
Rye flour, dark	1 cup	415	3.5/.4	1.5/.42	29	1.33	na	934	na	0	1
Rye flour, light	1 cup	374	1.4/.14	.58/.16	15	1	na	238	na	0	2
Rye flour, medium	1 cup	361	1.8/.2	.79/.21	15	1	na	347	na	0	3
Spelt flour	1 cup	440	4/0	na	8	na	na	na	na	0	na
Sunflower seed flour	1 cup	209	1/.08	.56/.16	3	22.9	na	43	high	0	2
Triticale flour	1 cup	439	2.4/.4	na	19	na	0	na	na	0	na
White flour, all-purpose, enriched	1 cup	455	1/.2	.52/.1	3.4	.34	0	134	na	0	3
White flour, cake	1 cup	496	1/.2	.52/.1	2.4	.42	0	144	na	0	3
White flour, self-rising, enriched	1 cup	442	1/.2	.51/.1	3.4	.27	0	155	na	0	1588
White flour, tortilla	1 cup	450	12/4.5	1.7/5	na	74.5	na	111	na	0	751
White flour, unbleached	1 cup	455	1/.2	.51/.1	3.4	.34	0	134	na	0	3
White rice flour	1 cup	578	2/6	.6/.7	4	.19	0	120	na	0	0
Whole wheat flour	1 cup	407	2/.4	.93/.28	15	.49	0	486	na	0	6

178

Food	Serving Size	Calories	Fat/Sat. Fat (gm)	Poly/Mono Fat (gm)	Fiber (gm)	Sugars (gm)	Carotenoids (mcg or mg)	Potassium (mg)	*Omega-3 Fat	Trans Fat	Sodium
Grains											
Barley, pearled, cooked	1 cup	193	.7/.15	.34/.09	6*SOL	.44	7 mcg (BC)	146	na	0	5
Basmati rice, cooked	1 cup	230	4/0	na	0	na	0	na	na	0	na
Brown rice, instant (Minute Rice)	1 cup	240	2/0	na	0	na	0	na	na	0	na
Brown rice, long-grain, cooked	1 cup	216	2/.35	.63/.84	3.5	.68	0	154	na	0	2
Brown rice, medium-grain, cooked	1 cup	218	1.6/.3	.58/.58	3.5	45.8	0	84	na	0	10
Brown rice, short-grain, cooked	1 cup	na	na	na	na	na	0	na	na	0	na
Brown rice, Spanish, cooked	1 cup	260	2.5/.5	na	5	na	na	na	na	0	na
Bulgur, cooked	1 cup	151	4/.07	.18/.06	8	.18	0	124	na	0	9
Corn bran	1 cup	170	.7/.1	.32/.18	65*SOL	0	na	33	na	0	5
Couscous, cooked	1 cup	176	.25/.05	.1/.03	2	.16	na	91	na	0	8
Couscous pilaf mix, cooked	1 cup	196	0/0	na	0	na	na	na	na	0	na
Millet, cooked	1 cup	207	2/3	4/2.6	2	na	na	na	na	0	na
Quinoa	1 cup	636	10/1	4/2.6	10	117	0	1258	na	0	36
Rye	1 cup	566	4/5	1.9/.5	25	1.76	na	466	na	0	10
Semolina	1 cup	601	1.75/.25	.71/2	6.5	121	na	311	na	0	2
Wheat Bran	¼ cup	30	.6/.09	.3/.09	7*SOL	.06	0	171	na	0	0

Food	Serving Size	Calories	Fat/Sat. Fat (gm)	Poly/Mono Fat (gm)	Fiber (gm)	Sugars (gm)	Carotenoids (mcg or mg)	Potassium (mg)	*Omega-3 Fat	Trans Fat	Sodium
Wheat germ	2 tbsp.	50	.3/.2	.82/.2	2*SOL	7.15	0	123	high	0	2
Wheat:											
Hard red	1 cup	632	4/.6	1.2/3.8	23	.79	0	697	na	0	4
Hard white	1 cup	657	3/.5	1.4/3.9	na	.79	0	829	na	0	4
Soft red	1 cup	556	2.6/.5	2.9/3	21	124	0	667	na	0	3
Soft white	1 cup	571	3/.6	1.4/3.38	21	.69	0	731	na	0	3
Sprouted	1 cup	214	1.4/.2	.29/.3	1	45.9	0	183	na	0	17
White rice, instant, cooked	1 cup	162	.3/.1	.6/.16	1	.08	0	.08	na	0	.07
White rice, long-grain, cooked w/salt	1 cup	205	.44/.12	.12/14	0	.08	0	55	na	0	604
White rice, medium-grain, cooked	1 cup	242	.4/.1	.1/.12	.6	58.9	0	53	na	0	0
White rice, short-grain, cooked	1 cup	242	.35/.09	.1/.1	na	33.2	0	54	na	0	0
White rice, Spanish or Mexican	1 cup	216	4/.6	na	3	na	689 mcg (BC)	na	na	0	na
Wild rice, cooked	1 cup	166	.6/.08	.35/.08	3	1.2	0	166	na	0	5
FRUITS											
Acerola cherries, raw	1 cup	31.4	.3/.1	na	1.1	na	453 mcg (BC)	na	na	0	na
Apple: Raw (3¼" diameter), with skin	1 fruit	81	.36/.1	.1/.01	4*SOL	22	41 mcg (AC)	227	na	0	2

Food	Serving Size	Calories	Fat/Sat. Fat (gm)	Poly/Mono Fat (gm)	Fiber (gm)	Sugars (gm)	Carotenoids (mcg or mg)	Potassium (mg)	*Omega-3 Fat	Trans Fat	Sodium
Raw (3/4" diameter), no skin	1 fruit	63	.34/t	.04/t	2*SOL	12.9	41 mcg (BC)	115	na	0	0
Dried	5 pieces	78	.1/t	.03/t	3*SOL	18.3	na	144	na	0	28
Applesauce, w/o salt, sweetened	1 cup	194	.5/.1	.14/.02	3*SOL	42	16 mcg (BC)	156	na	0	8
Applesauce, w/o salt unsweetened	1 cup	105	.1/0	.03/t	3*SOL	24.6	44 mcg (BC)	183	na	0	5
Apricots:											
Raw	1 fruit	17	.14/0	.03/.06	.9	3.23	894 mcg (BC)	91	na	0	0
Canned, heavy syrup	1 cup	214	.21/0	.04/.08	4	51.3	2 mg (BC)	361	na	0	10
Canned, juice pack	1 cup	117	.1/0	.02/.04	4	26.2	2.5 mg (BC)	403	na	0	10
Canned, light syrup	1 cup	159	.1/0	.02/.05	4	37.7	2 mg (BC)	349	na	0	10
Canned, water pack	1 cup	66	.4/0	.07/.17	4	11.6	1.5 mg (BC)	467	na	0	17
Dried	10 halves	83	.16/0	.02/.17	3	18.6	1.5 mg (BC)	390	na	0	14
Avocado, California	1 ea.	278	26.5/4.2	3.1/17	8.7	.52	663 mcg (BC)	877	na	0	14
Avocado, Florida	1 ea.	489	30.7/4	5/17	15	7.4	1.1 mg (BC)	1067	na	0	6
Banana (8" long)	1 fruit	109	.57/.2	.1/.04	3*SOL	16.6	56 mcg (BC)	487	na	0	1
Banana chips, dried	10 chips	51	9.7	.06/.2	.9*SOL	3.5	23 mcg (BC)	53	na	0	1
Blackberries, raw	1 cup	75	.56/0	0/.07	7.6	7	138 mcg (BC)	233	na	0	1
Blueberries:											
Raw	1 cup	81	.55/0	.2/.07	4	14.4	87 mcg (BC)	112	na	0	1
Frozen, sweetened	1 cup	186	.3/0	.13/t	5	45	55 mcg (BC)	138	na	0	2
Frozen, unsweetened	1 cup	79	1/0	.43/.14	4.2	13	46 mcg (AC)	84	na	0	2

Food	Serving Size	Calories	Fat/Sat. Fat (gm)	Poly/Mono Fat (gm)	Fiber (gm)	Sugars (gm)	Carotenoids (mcg or mg)	Potassium (mg)	*Omega-3 Fat	Trans Fat	Sodium
Cherries, raw	10 cherries	49	0/0	0/0	1.5	13	518 mcg (BC)	268	na	0	5
Cherries, water pack	1 cup	114	.3/.1	.09/.08	2.7	25.4	238 mcg (BC)	325	na	0	2
Cranberries, raw	1 cup	46	.2/0	.05/.02	4	3.8	29 mcg (BC)	81	na	0	2
Currants, black	1 cup	123	t/0	t/t	5.4	17.2	80 mcg (BC)	361	na	0	2
Currants, red	1 cup	67	t/0	t/t	4.5	8.25	80 mcg (BC)	308	na	0	1
Dates, whole without pits	5 dates	114	.19/t	t/t	3	79.76	14 mcg (BC)	835	na	0	4
Dates, chopped	1 cup	490	1/t	.03/.06	13	112.8	na	1168	na	0	1
Figs, dried	2 figs	42	.16/.02	.06/.03	4.6	8	30 mcg (BC)	114	na	0	2
Figs, canned, light syrup	1 cup	174	.3/.1	.12/.05	4.5	46.7	60 mcg (BC)	257	na	0	3
Fruit cocktail, heavy syrup	1 cup	181	.17/0	.08/.03	2.5*SOL	44.4	298 mcg (BC)	218	na	0	15
Fruit cocktail, juice pack	1 cup	109	.02/0	t/t	2.4*SOL	25.7	441 mcg (BC)	225	na	0	9
Fruit cocktail, light syrup	1 cup	140	.2/0	.07/.03	2.4*SOL	33.7	305 mcg (BC)	215	na	0	15
Fruit cocktail, water pack	1 cup	39.4	.1/0	.05/.02	1.2*SOL	17.8	185 mcg (BC)	223	na	0	9
Grapefruit: Pink (3¾" diameter)	1 half	37	.12/0	.02/.01	1.3*SOL	9	741 mcg (BC) 1.8 mg (LYC)	159	na	0	1
White (3¾" diameter)	1 half	39	.12/0	.02/.01	1.3*SOL	9	741 mcg (BC) 1.8 mg (LYC)	159	na	0	1

182

Food	Serving Size	Calories	Fat/Sat. Fat (gm)	Poly/Mono Fat (gm)	Fiber (gm)	Sugars (gm)	Carotenoids (mcg or mg)	Potassium (mg)	*Omega-3 Fat	Trans Fat	Sodium
Canned sections, light syrup	1 cup	152	.25/0	.06/.03	1*SOL	38	0	328	na	0	5
Canned sections, water pack	1 cup	88	.2/0	.06/.03	1*SOL	21	0	322	na	0	5
Grapes, red	1 cup	114	.93/.3	.08/t	1.6	24.8	67 mcg (BC)	306	na	0	3
Grapes, white	1 cup	114	.93/.3	.08/t	1.6	24.8	67 mcg (BC)	306	na	0	3
Guava	1 medium	46	.5/.2	.2/.05	5	4.9	427 mcg (BC)	229	na	0	1
Kiwi fruit, raw	1 fruit	46	2.6/0	.2/.04	2.6	6.8	82 mcg (BC)	237	na	0	2
Lemon, raw, without peel	1 fruit	17	1.6/0	.05/t	1.6*SOL	1.4	10mcg (BC)	80	na	0	1
Mango, diced	1 cup	107	.45/.1	.08/.17	3	24.4	3.8 mg (BC)	257	na	0	3
Melons:											
Cantaloupe	½ melon	24	.19/0	.13/t	.55	12	1.3 mg (BC)	417	na	0	25
Casaba	1 cup	44	.2/0	.07/t	1.4	9.7	31 mcg (BC)	309	na	0	na
Honeydew	½ melon	56	.2/0	.07/t	1	19	38 mcg (BC)	285	na	0	23
Nectarine (2½" diameter)	1 fruit	67	.63/.1	.15/.12	2*SOL	10.7	604 mcg (BC)	273	na	0	0
Orange, medium	1 fruit	62	.16/0	.03/.11	3*SOL	12	165 mcg (BC) 160 mcg (BCR) 245 mcg (LU+Z)	237	na	0	0
Orange sections, canned, juice pack	1 cup	93	.3/0	na	3.4*SOL	na	236 mcg (BC)	na	na	0	na
Orange sections, raw	1 cup	85	.22/0	.04/.11	4*SOL	16.8	na	326	na	0	0
Papaya, diced	1 cup	55	.2/t	.04/.05	2.5	8.3	386 mcg (BC) 1 mg (BCR)	360	na	0	4

Food	Serving Size	Calories	Fat/Sat. Fat (gm)	Poly/Mono Fat (gm)	Fiber (gm)	Sugars (gm)	Carotenoids (mcg or mg)	Potassium (mg)	*Omega-3 Fat	Trans Fat	Sodium
Papaya, whole	1 fruit	119	.43/t	.09/.1	5.5	17.9	510 mcg (BC)	781	na	0	9
Passion fruit	1 fruit	18	.1/0	na	2	na	76 mcg (BC)	na	na	0	na
Peaches:											
Raw, medium	1 fruit	42	.25/.02	.08/.07	2	8.2	317 mcg (BC)	186	na	0	0
Canned, heavy syrup	1 cup	194	.26/t	.1/.09	3.4	45.4	875 mcg (BC)	206	na	0	10
Canned, juice pack	1 cup	109	.07/0	.04/.03	3	26	570 mcg (BC)	320	na	0	10
Canned, water pack	1 cup	59	.1/0	.07/.05	3	11.7	776 mcg (BC)	242	na	0	7
Dried	3 halves	93	.3/0	.15/.11	3	21.9	518 mcg (BC)	413	na	0	3
Frozen, sliced, sweetened	1 cup	235	.3/0	.16/.12	4.5	55	420 mcg (BC)	325	na	0	15
Frozen, sliced	1 cup	107	.2/0	na	5	na	767 mcg (BC)	na	na	0	na
Pears:											
Raw, medium	1 fruit	98	.66/0	.05/.04	4*SOL	16	45 mcg (BC)	198	na	0	2
Canned, heavy syrup	1 cup	197	.35/0	.08/.07	4*SOL	40.4	3 mcg (BC)	173	na	0	13
Canned, juice pack	1 cup	124	.17/0	.04/.03	4*SOL	24	14 mcg (BC)	238	na	0	10
Canned, water pack	1 cup	71	.1/0	.02/.03	4*SOL	15	0	129	na	0	5
Dried	10 ea.	459	1/t	.3/.24	13*SOL	104	na	987	na	0	11
Persimmons, medium	1 fruit	67	0/0	0/0	3.6	21	1.2 mg (BC) 1.5 mg (BCR) 834 mcg (LU+Z)	270	na	0	2
Pineapple:											
Fresh chunks	1 cup	76	.67/0	.06/.02	2*SOL	8.4	19 mcg (BC)	178	na	0	2
Canned, heavy syrup	1 cup	195	.3/0	.1/.03	3*SOL	42.9	15 mcg (BC)	264	na	0	3
Canned, juice pack	1 cup	150	.2/0	.07/.02	2*SOL	36	60 mcg (BC)	304	na	0	2

Food	Serving Size	Calories	Fat/Sat. Fat (gm)	Poly/Mono Fat (gm)	Fiber (gm)	Sugars (gm)	Carotenoids (mcg or mg)	Potassium (mg)	*Omega-3 Fat	Trans Fat	Sodium
Canned, light syrup	1 cup	131	3/0	.1/.03	2*SOL	31.9	15 mcg (BC)	265	na	0	3
Canned, water pack	1 cup	79	.2/0	.08/.03	2*SOL	18.4	30 mcg (BC)	312	na	0	2
Plantains, raw	1 fruit	218	.66/t	.1/.06	4*SOL	26.8	na	893	na	0	7
Plantains, cooked	1 cup	176	.28/t	.05/.02	3.5*SOL	21.6	na	716	na	0	8
Plums:											
Raw, medium	1 fruit	36	.41/0	.03/.09	1	6.5	127 mcg (BC)	104	na	0	0
Canned, heavy syrup	1 cup	230	.26/0	.05/.16	2.5	39.5	403 mcg (BC)	170	na	0	35
Canned, juice pack	1 cup	146	.05/0	.01/.03	2.5	35.8	1.5 mg (BC)	388	na	0	3
Canned, light syrup	1 cup	159	.3/0	.06/.17	2.5	38.7	393 mcg (BC)	234	na	0	50
Canned, water pack	1 cup	102	0/0	0/0	2.5	25	1.4 mg (BC)	314	na	0	2
Pomegranate, raw	1 fruit	105	.5/.1	.1/.07	.9	25.5	0	399	na	0	5
Prunes:											
Dried, pitted, uncooked	5 prunes	100	.22/0	.03/.02	3	16	502 mcg (BC)	307	na	0	1
Stewed	1 cup	265	.57/0	.15/.45	16	83	461 mcg (BC)	988	na	0	6
Raisins	1 packet	42	.06/t	t/t	na	8.3	na	105	na	0	2
Raspberries:											
Raw	1 cup	60	.68/0	.38/.06	8	4.4	15 mcg (AC) 96 mcg (BC)	151	na	0	1
Frozen, sweetened	1 cup	258	.4/0	.2/.04	11	54.4	90 mcg (BC)	285	na	0	3
Frozen, unsweetened	1 cup	123	1.4/0	na	17	na	185 mcg (BC)	na	na	0	na
Rhubarb, canned, light syrup	1 cup	220	.2/.1	na	3.5	na	120 mcg (BC)	na	na	0	na
Rhubarb, cooked	1 cup	278	.5/.1	na	4	na	108 mcg (BC)	na	na	0	na

Food	Serving Size	Calories	Fat/Sat. Fat (gm)	Poly/Mono Fat (gm)	Fiber (gm)	Sugars (gm)	Carotenoids (mcg or mg)	Potassium (mg)	*Omega-3 Fat	Trans Fat	Sodium
Strawberries:											
Raw	1 cup	50	.6l/0	.26/.07	4	3.3	8 mcg (AC) 30 mcg (BC)	254	na	0	2
Frozen, sweetened	1 cup	222	.33/0	.1/.03	5	10	38 mcg (BC)	327	na	0	4
Frozen, unsweetened	1 cup.	77	.2/0	.16/.05	5	61	53 mcg (BC)	250	na	0	8
Tangelo	1 fruit	45	.1/0	na	2.3*SOL	na	120 mcg (BC)	na	na	0	na
Tangerine, medium	1	37	.16/0	.05/.11	2*SOL	8.9	464 mcg (BC) 407 mcg (BCR) 204 mcg (LU+Z)	139	na	0	2
Tangerine (mandarin), canned light syrup	1 cup	154	.25/0	.05/.04	1.7*SOL	39	1.3 mg (BC)	197	na	0	15
Tangerine (mandarin), juice pack	1 cup	92	.1/0	.01/.11	1.7*SOL	22	1.3 mg (BC)	331	na	0	12
Watermelon, wedge	1	92	1/.1	.1/.1	1.4	17.7	844 mcg (BC) 14 mg (LYC)	320	na	0	3
GOOSE											
Roasted:											
Meat and skin	1 cup	427	31/10	3.5/14	0	0	0	461	na	0	98
Meat only	1 cup	340	18/6.5	2/6	0	0	0	555	na	0	109
Pate	1 tbsp.	60	5.7/1.8	3.3/1.9	0	.61	0	18	na	0	91
GRANOLA BARS											
Chewy	1 bar	126	5/2	1.5/1	1.3	18.8	na	91	na	+	78

Food	Serving Size	Calories	Fat/Sat. Fat (gm)	Poly/Mono Fat (gm)	Fiber (gm)	Sugars (gm)	Carotenoids (mcg or mg)	Potassium (mg)	*Omega-3 Fat	Trans Fat	Sodium
Chewy w/chocolate chips (Quaker Oats)	1 bar	127	5/4	na	1	na	2 mcg (BC)	na	na	+	na
Chewy w/coconut	1 bar	195	7.6/5.5	.7/.8	1	11.8	2.4 mcg (BC)	140	na	+	120
Chocolate coated (Quaker Oats)	1 bar	130	6/3	na	1	na	2.4 mcg (BC)	na	na	+	na
Choclate coated (Sweet Success)	1 bar	153	7/3	na	1	na	3 mcg (BC)	na	na	+	na
Chocolate coated, w/nuts	1 bar	178	11/6	.7/2.4	1	19.7	2.4 mcg (BC)	125	high	+	71
Coconut, chocolate coated	1 bar	198	13/9	na	2.4	na	5 mcg (BC)	na	na	+	na
Fruit and nut, low fat (Nature Valley)	1 bar	106	2/2	na	1.5	na	284 mcg (BC)	na	na	0	na
Fruit, nuts, and oats, lowfat (Kellogg's)	1 bar	80	1/.2	na	1	na	213 mcg (BC)	na	na	+	na
Non-chocolate coating (Quaker Oats)	1 bar	131	6/1	na	1	na	t (BC)	na	na	+	na
Nonfat (Health Valley) Fat-Free	1 bar	142	.4/.1	na	3	na	129 mcg (BC)	na	na	0	na
Nougat (Nature Valley Granola Cluster)	1 bar	138	4.5/2	na	1.4	na	2.4 mcg (BC)	na	na	0	na
Peanut butter (Nature Valley)	1 bar	90	3/.5	na	1	na	na	na	na	0	na

Food	Serving Size	Calories	Fat/Sat. Fat (gm)	Poly/Mono Fat (gm)	Fiber (gm)	Sugars (gm)	Carotenoids (mcg or mg)	Potassium (mg)	*Omega-3 Fat	Trans Fat	Sodium
Peanuts and wheat germ	1 bar	206	9/1	na	2	na	8 mcg (BC)	na	na	un	na
Plain	1 bar	115	5/6	3.4/1.2	1.3	18	na	94	na	un	82
Rice-based (Kellogg's Rice Krispies bar)	1 bar	119	5/1.5	na	1	na	0	na	na	+	na
Trail mix chewy (Quaker)	1 bar	130	5/0	na	t	na	na	na	na	+	na
Yogurt coated	1 bar	96	3/1	na	2.2	na	t (BC)	na	na	un	na
HOT DOGS											
Beef	1	185	17/7	.5/7.4	0	1.8	0	76	na	0	600
Beef and pork	1	189	17/6	1.5/7.8	0	0	0	95	na	0	638
Beef, lowfat	1	136	11/5	.3/4	0	0	0	125	na	0	455
Beef and pork, fat free	1	92	6/2	.5/.25	0	0	0	86	na	0	716
Chicken	1	150	11/3	1.8/3.8	0	0	0	38	na	0	617
Chicken, beef, and pork	1	175	15/5	na	0	na	0	na	na	0	na
Light (Oscar Mayer)	1	110	8/3.5	.57/4.3	0	1.2	0	229	na	0	615
Meat and poultry, fat-free (Ballpark or Oscar Mayer)	1	40	0/0	0/0	0	1.9	0	234	na	0	464
Meat and poultry, lowfat (Healthy Choice)	1	72	1.6/.6	na	0	na	0	na	na	0	na

Food	Serving Size	Calories	Fat/Sat. Fat (gm)	Poly/Mono Fat (gm)	Fiber (gm)	Sugars (gm)	Carotenoids (mcg or mg)	Potassium (mg)	*Omega-3 Fat	Trans Fat	Sodium
Meatless	1	140	7/1	5.5/2.7	0	0	0	69	na	0	330
Pork, light (Oscar Mayer)	1	111	8.5/3	1.2/3.8	0	.86	0	226	na	0	591
Pork and turkey (Oscar Mayer)	1	145	13/4	1.9/6.2	0	.81	0	73	na	0	445
3% fat (Hormel)	1	45	1/0	na	0	na	0	na	na	0	na
Turkey	1	132	10/3.4	2.5/2.5	0	0	0	81	na	0	642
Turkey and chicken (Louis Rich)	1	85	6/2	1.4/2.5	0	.68	0	72	na	0	511
ICE CREAM & FROZEN DESSERTS (REDUCED FAT)											
Creamsicle (Carbsmart)	1 bar	20	1/1	na	0	0	na	na	na	0	0
Fudge bar (Healthy Choice)	1 bar	80	1/.5	na	0	2	na	200	na	0	60
Fudge bar (Skinny Cow)	1 bar	100	0/0	na	1	1	na	na	na	0	70
Fudge bar (Weight Watchers)	1 bar	10	1/.5	na	5	16	na	260	na	0	70
Ice cream bar, Cookies & Cream (Weight Watchers)	1 bar	140	5/1.5	na	4	14	na	na	na	0	95
Ice cream bar, Sundae (Weight Watchers)	1 bar	140	4/3	na	4	14	na	na	na	0	85

Food	Serving Size	Calories	Fat/Sat. Fat (gm)	Poly/Mono Fat (gm)	Fiber (gm)	Sugars (gm)	Carotenoids (mcg or mg)	Potassium (mg)	*Omega-3 Fat	Trans Fat	Sodium
Ice cream bar, low fat mocha swirl (Healthy Choice)	1 bar	90	1.5/1	na	1	14	na	na	na	0	50
Ice cream bar, strawberry (Healthy Choice)	1 bar	90	1/.5	na	1	13	na	na	na	0	40
Ice cream sandwich, chocolate (Weight Watchers)	1 sandwich	140	2/1	na	4	13	na	150	na	0	140
Ice cream sandwich, Vanilla (Weight Watchers)	1 sandwich	140	2/.5	na	4	12	na	105	na	0	140
Klondike, Fat Free Chocolate	1 bar	130	1.5/0	na	3	14	na	na	na	0	120
Klondike, Fat Free Vanilla	1 bar	130	1.5/0	na	3	14	na	na	na	0	120
Klondike, Vanilla, Carbsmart	1 bar	170	15/11	na	2	5	na	na	na	0	40
Fruit bar, frozen, nonfat orange (Tropical Swirls)	1 bar	60	2/1	na	1	3	na	na	na	0	30
Fruit bar, frozen, nonfat, rasp (Tropical Swirls)	1 bar	60	2/1	na	1	3	2.4 mcg (BC)	na	na	0	35

190

Food	Serving Size	Calories	Fat/Sat. Fat (gm)	Poly/Mono Fat (gm)	Fiber (gm)	Sugars (gm)	Carotenoids (mcg or mg)	Potassium (mg)	*Omega-3 Fat	Trans Fat	Sodium
Ice cream, chocolate (Healthy Choice)	4 oz.	130	2/1	na	1	17	4 mcg (BC)	na	na	0	70
Ice cream, peanut butter cup, low fat (Healthy Choice)	½ cup	120	2/1	na	1	17	na	na	na	0	70
Ice cream, vanilla (Healthy Choice)	4 oz.	120	2/1	na	1	17	0	na	na	0	70

LAMB

Food	Serving Size	Calories	Fat/Sat. Fat (gm)	Poly/Mono Fat (gm)	Fiber (gm)	Sugars (gm)	Carotenoids (mcg or mg)	Potassium (mg)	*Omega-3 Fat	Trans Fat	Sodium
Chop	1 medium chop	345	27/12	na	0	0	0	na	na	0	na
Leg, roasted	3 oz.	199	12/6	.47/4.7	0	0	0	266	na	0	57
Rib, roasted	3 oz.	290	23/10	1.7/9.8	0	0	0	235	na	0	63
Shoulder, roasted	3 oz.	241	16.3/6.8	1.3/6.6	0	0	0	211	na	0	57
Sweetbreads	3 oz.	148	3.6/1.3	na	0	0	0	na	na	0	na

MILK & MILK BEVERAGES

Food	Serving Size	Calories	Fat/Sat. Fat (gm)	Poly/Mono Fat (gm)	Fiber (gm)	Sugars (gm)	Carotenoids (mcg or mg)	Potassium (mg)	*Omega-3 Fat	Trans Fat	Sodium
Buttermilk, cultured	1 cup	90	1/0	.02/.2	0	1.6	0	55	na	0	26
Chocolate milk:											
1%	1 cup	158	2.5/1.5	.04/.7	1.25	25	0	423	na	0	150
2%	1 cup	190	5/0	1.5/3	0	25	0	458	na	0	154
Whole	1 cup	210	8/0	.49/2	0	31.7	0	418	na	0	150
Milk:											
Instant nonfat (dried), prepared	1 cup	80	0/0	0/0	0	12	0	389	na	0	125

Food	Serving Size	Calories	Fat/Sat Fat (gm)	Poly/Mono Fat (gm)	Fiber (gm)	Sugars (gm)	Carotenoids (mcg or mg)	Potassium (mg)	*Omega-3 Fat	Trans Fat	Sodium
Lowfat (1%)	1 cup	100–104	2/1.5	.08/7	0	11.8	0	407	na	0	127
Nonfat	1 cup	90	.6/.4	t/.2	0	12.7	0	366	na	0	107
Reduced fat (2%)	1 cup	121	4.6/1.3	.2/1.4	0	12.3	0	366	na	0	100
Whole	1 cup	150	8/5	.5/2	0	12.8	0	349	na	0	98
Milk, evaporated:											
Low-fat (Carnation)	½ cup	110	3/2	na	0	na	0	na	na	0	na
Regular (Carnation)	½ cup	170	10/0	na	0	na	0	na	na	0	na
Milk, goat's	1 cup	168	10/3	.4/2.7	0	11	0	498	na	0	122
Sweetened, condensed	1 fl. oz.	123	3.3/2	.1/.9	0	20	0	142	na	0	49
Milk Beverages:											
Eggnog, nonalcoholic	1 cup	350	17/0	.9/5.7	0	137	0	419	na	0	137
Hot cocoa, prepared with water (Swiss Miss)	1 packet	110	3/1.3	na	0	102	0	94	na	0	102
Hot cocoa, prepared with water, sugar free (Nestle)	1 packet	55	.43/.01	.1/.8	.36	142	0	288	na	0	142
Instant Breakfast, with 2% milk	1 packet	131	7.3/.2	.1/.1	na	142	0	350	na	0	142
Instant Breakfast, with 2% milk, sugar free	1 packet	72	1/.4	.2/.4	na	143	0	341	na	0	143
Malted milk, fortified, prepared with whole milk	1 cup	225	9/5.5	.56/.2	.27	191	0	530	na	0	191

Food	Serving Size	Calories	Fat/Sat. Fat (gm)	Poly/Mono Fat (gm)	Fiber (gm)	Sugars (gm)	Carotenoids (mcg or mg)	Potassium (mg)	*Omega-3 Fat	Trans Fat	Sodium
Milkshake, chocolate	11 oz.	356	8/5	.3/19	.9	347	0	700	na	un	347
Milkshake, vanilla	11 oz.	350	9.5/6	.35/2.7	0	297	0	573	na	un	297

NUTS, SEEDS & PRODUCTS

Almonds:

Food	Serving Size	Calories	Fat/Sat. Fat (gm)	Poly/Mono Fat (gm)	Fiber (gm)	Sugars (gm)	Carotenoids (mcg or mg)	Potassium (mg)	*Omega-3 Fat	Trans Fat	Sodium
Butter	1 tbsp.	101	9.5/.9	na	.6	na	0	na	high	0	na
Dry roasted, salted	22 nuts (1 oz.)	169	15/1	3.6/9.5	3.4	1.3	0	211	high	0	96
Oil roasted, salted	22 nuts (1 oz.)	172	16/1.2	3.8/9.7	3	1.3	0	198	high	0	96
Slivered	1 cup	624	55/4	13/34	13	5.2	0	786	high	0	1
Brazil nuts	6–8 nuts	186	19/5	5.8/6.9	1.5	.66	0	187	high	0	1
Cashews:											
Butter	1 tbsp.	94	8/1.6	1.3/4.7	.32	.8	0	87	high	0	98
Dry roasted, salted	18 nuts (1 oz.)	163	13/2.6	2.2/7.7	.85	1.4	0	160	high	0	181
Oil roasted, salted	18 nuts (1 oz.)	164	14/3	2.4/7.3	1	1.4	0	179	high	0	87
Chestnuts	10 nuts	206	2/3	.28/.6	4.3	49	10 mcg (BC)	447	high	0	3
Coconut:											
2 x 2 x ½"	1 piece	159	15/13	.16/6	4	2.8	0	160	high	0	9
Shredded, sweetened	1 oz.	135	9/8	na	1.2	na	0	na	high	0	na
Shredded, unsweetened	1 oz.	187	18/16	na	4.6	na	0	na	high	0	na
Flaxseed	1 tbsp.	59	4/4	2.7/.8	3.4	.13	0	82	high	0	4
Hazelnuts	10 nuts	88	8.5/.6	1/6.4	1.4	.6	6.6 mcg (BC)	95	high	0	0

Food	Serving Size	Calories	Fat/Sat. Fat (gm)	Poly/Mono Fat (gm)	Fiber (gm)	Sugars (gm)	Carotenoids (mcg or mg)	Potassium (mg)	*Omega-3 Fat	Trans Fat	Sodium
Macadamia nuts:											
Dry roasted, salted	10–12 nuts (1 oz.)	203	22/4	.4/16.8	2.3	1.17	1.8 mcg (BC)	103	high	0	75
Mixed nuts:											
Dry roasted, salted	1 oz.	168	15/2	3/8.9	2.5	1.32	1.8 mcg (BC)	169	high	0	190
Oil roasted, salted	1 oz.	174	16/2.6	3.8/9	1.6	1.2	3.6 mcg (BC)	165	high	0	119
Peanuts:											
Boiled	About 30 nuts (1 oz.)	89	6/9	1.9/3	2.5	.69	0	50	high	0	210
Dry roasted, salted	1 oz.	166	14/2	4.4/6.8	2.3	1	0	187	high	0	230
Honey roasted	1 oz.	153	12/2	na	2.3	4.9	0	na	high	0	na
Oil roasted	1 oz.	163	14/2	4/7	2.6	1	0	196	high	0	86
Spanish, oil roasted	1 oz.	164	14/2	4.8/6.2	2.5	1	0	220	high	0	123
Peanut butter:											
Chunky, w/o salt	2 tbsp.	188.5	16/3	4.7/7.9	na	2.7	33 mg	238	high	un	5
Reduced fat	2 tbsp.	187	12/2.6	3.6/5.6	na	2.7	na	234	high	un	189
Smooth	2 tbsp.	190	16/3	4.4/7.6	na	2.9	33 mg	208	high	un	147
Pecans:											
Dried	20 halves (1 oz.)	196	20/2	6/11.5	3	1.1	22 mcg (BC)	116	high	0	0
Dry roasted, salted	20 halves (1 oz.)	201	21/1.8	5.8/12	2.7	1.1	22 mcg (BC)	120	high	0	109
Oil roasted, salted	15 halves (1 oz.)	203	21/2	6.7/11	2.7	1.1	na	111	high	0	111

Food	Serving Size	Calories	Fat/Sat. Fat (gm)	Poly/Mono Fat (gm)	Fiber (gm)	Sugars (gm)	Carotenoids (mcg or mg)	Potassium (mg)	*Omega-3 Fat	Trans Fat	Sodium
Pine nuts	10 nuts	6	1.2/.09	.6/.3	.1	.06	.6 mcg (BC)	11	high	0	0
Pistachios, dry roasted	47 nuts (1 oz.)	161	13/1.6	3.9/6.9	3	2.2	40 mcg (BC)	295	high	0	115
Pumpkin seeds, dried	1 oz.	146	12/2	5.4/3.7	1	.65	64 mcg (BC)	229	high	0	163
Sesame seeds, dry	1 tbsp.	47	4.4/.6	1.9/1.6	1	.04	t	33	high	0	2
Sunflower seeds, hulled:											
Dry roasted	1 oz.	93	8/.8	9.3/2.7	1.4	.77	0	241	high	0	116
Oil roasted	1 oz.	105	10/1	9.7/2.3	1.2	.88	5.4 mcg (BC)	137	high	0	116
Tahini (sesame butter)	1 tbsp.	85.5	7/1	3.5/3	1.4	3	6.6 mcg (BC)	69	high	0	5
Trail Mix:											
Regular	1 cup	693	44/8	14/8.8	9	67.3	11 mcg (BC)	518	high	un	1028
With chocolate chips	1 cup	707	47/9	16/19.8	na	65.6	na	946	high	un	177
Tropical	1 cup	570	24/12	7/3.5	na	91.8	na	993	high	un	14
Walnuts:											
Black	14 halves (1 oz.)	172	16/1	10/4	1.4	.31	20 mcg (BC)	148	high	0	1
English	14 halves (1 oz.)	185	18.5/1.7	13/2.5	2	.74	20 mcg (BC)	125	high	0	1
PANCAKES, WAFFLES & FRENCH TOAST											
French toast, from recipe, w/2% milk	1 slice	149	7/1.7	1.7/2.9	na	16.2	na	87	na	un	311
French toast, ready-to-heat	1 piece	126	3.6/.9	.7/1.2	.65	18.9	1.2 mcg	79	na	+	292

195

Food	Serving Size	Calories	Fat/Sat. Fat (gm)	Poly/Mono Fat (gm)	Fiber (gm)	Sugars (gm)	Carotenoids (mcg or mg)	Potassium (mg)	*Omega-3 Fat	Trans Fat	Sodium
Pancakes:											
Blueberry	1 pancake, 6" dia.	105	3.5/1	3.2/1.8	1	22.3	10 mcg	106	na	un	317
Buckwheat	1 pancake, 6" dia.	98	3.5/1	.2/.1	1.4	2	3.6 mcg	90	na	un	393
Buttermilk, Eggo's (Kellogg's)	1 serving	233	6.7/1.4	na	1	na	na	na	na	+	na
Buttermilk, from recipe	1 pancake, 6" dia.	175	7/1.4	3.4/1.8	na	22	na	112	na	un	402
Plain	1 pancake, 6" dia.	126	1.8/.4	.4/.5	1	31.8	9 mcg	53	na	un	372
Cornmeal	1 pancake, 6" dia.	112	3.3/.8	na	1	na	55 mcg	na	na	un	na
Plain, ready-to-heat, from frozen	1 pancake, 6" dia.	167	2.4/.5	.7/.8	1.3	20.2	na	97	na	un	344
Reduced calorie	1 pancake, 6" dia.	99	.4/.06	.2/.08	4.4	20.9	6.6 mcg	192	na	un	129
Rye	1 pancake, 6" dia.	165	6/1.3	na	2	na	1.2 mcg	na	na	un	na
Sourdough	1 pancake, 6" dia.	121	3.6/.7	na	.8	na	0	na	na	un	na
Whole wheat	1 pancake, 6" dia.	127	5.6/1.2	3/2.1	2	38	4 mcg	360	na	un	738

196

Food	Serving Size	Calories	Fat/Sat. Fat (gm)	Poly/Mono Fat (gm)	Fiber (gm)	Sugars (gm)	Carotenoids (mcg or mg)	Potassium (mg)	*Omega-3 Fat	Trans Fat	Sodium
Waffles:											
Banana bread, Nutri-Grain (Kellogg's)	1 serving	212	7.4/1.3	1.9/4	2*SOL	5.2	na	140	high	+	280
Blueberry, Eggo (Kellogg's)	1 serving	73	1/.14	.3/.4	1	3	0	24	na	+	207
Frozen (Aunt Jemima)	1 serving	197	6/1.6	na	na	30.4	0	na	na	+	563
Golden Oat, Eggo (Kellogg's)	1 serving	137	2.2/.4	.7/.7	2.5*SOL	2.4	0	134	na	+	270
Lowfat, Eggo (Kellogg's)	1 serving	165	2.5/.6	.7/.7	.7	2	0	100	na	+	309
Nutri-Grain, Eggo (Kellogg's)	1 serving	142	2.2/.3	.7/.9	2.6*SOL	4	0	50	high	+	430
Plain, fat-free	1 serving	74	.1/0	na	.4	na	0	na	na	0	na
Plain, lowfat (Aunt Jemima)	1 serving	87	.7/.1	na	.4	na	0	na	na	0	na
Plain, from recipe	1 waffle, 7" dia.	218	11/2	5/2.6	na	24.7	0	119	na	un	383
Plain, ready-to-heat, from frozen	1 waffle, 4" sq.	88	3/.5	1/1.2	.8	1.4	0	48	na	un	292
Toaster	1 waffle, 4" sq.	87	2.7/.5	.9/1	.8	1.3	0	42	na	un	260

PASTA & NOODLES (COOKED)

Food	Serving Size	Calories	Fat/Sat. Fat (gm)	Poly/Mono Fat (gm)	Fiber (gm)	Sugars (gm)	Carotenoids (mcg or mg)	Potassium (mg)	*Omega-3 Fat	Trans Fat	Sodium
Chinese noodles, chow mein	1 cup	237	14/2	7.8/3.5	2	.12	0	54	na	0	198
Corn-based pasta	1 cup	176	1/.14	.4/.3	7	39	42 mcg	43	na	0	0
Egg noodle, enriched	1 cup	213	2.4/.5	.6/.7	2	.51	0	45	na	0	11
Egg noodle, spinach, enriched	1 cup	211	2.5/.6	.6/.8	3.7	.64	na	59	na	0	19
Japanese noodle, soba	1 cup	113	.1/.02	.03/.03	na	.24	na	40	na	0	68
Japanese noodle, somen	1 cup	231	.3/.04	.04/.04	na	48	na	51	na	0	283
Macaroni, elbow	1 cup	197	1/.3	.4/.1	2	.91	0	43	na	0	1
Macaroni, spinach	1 cup	191	.8/.1	na	5.4	na	44 mcg	na	na	0	na
Macaroni, vegetable	1 cup	171	.15/.02	.06/.02	6	1.1	na	42	na	0	8
Macaroni, elbows, whole wheat	1 cup	174	.75/.14	.3/.1	4	1.1	0	62	na	0	4
Pasta, fresh	1 cup	262	2/.3	.8/.2	na	49.8	0	48	na	0	12
Pasta, fresh, spinach	1 cup	260	2/.4	.4/.6	na	59	na	74	na	0	12
Pasta, linguini	1 cup	197	.9/.1	na	2.4	na	0	na	na	0	na
Rice noodles	1 cup	192	.35/.04	.04/.05	2	43.8	0	7	na	0	33
Spaghetti, enriched	1 cup	197	1/.1	.4/.01	3	.9	0	43	na	0	140
Spaghetti, enriched, spinach	1 cup	182	.9/.12	.4/.1	na	36.6	na	81	high	0	20
Spaghetti, enriched, whole wheat	1 cup	174	.75/.14	.3/.1	6	1.1	0	62	na	0	4

Food	Serving Size	Calories	Fat/Sat. Fat (gm)	Poly/Mono Fat (gm)	Fiber (gm)	Sugars (gm)	Carotenoids (mcg or mg)	Potassium (mg)	*Omega-3 Fat	Trans Fat	Sodium
PORK											
Boneless	3 oz.	149	7.6/1.7	.7/2.9	0	0	0	292	na	0	1155
Canned, extra lean	3 oz.	142	7/2.4	.1/.6	0	0	0	103	na	0	356
Patty, grilled	1 patty	203	18/6.7	.4/6	0	0	0	234	na	0	58
Roasted, lean portion	3 oz.	206	14/5	1.5/6.7	0	0	0	243	na	0	1009
Center rib, broiled	3 oz.	224	13/4.8	1/5.8	0	0	0	341	na	0	53
Chop, lean, breaded or floured, broiled or baked	1 med. (5.5 oz)	207	8.4/3	na	0	0	94 mcg	na	na	0	na
Chop, lean, broiled or baked	1 med. (5.5 oz.)	176	8/3	.7/3.8	0	0	0	236	na	0	50
Cutlet, lean, broiled or baked	3 oz.	181	9/3	na	0	0	0	na	na	0	na
Ground patty	1 patty	297	21/8	2.6/10	0	0	0	348	na	0	85
Roast, lean, loin	3 oz.	122	5/1.7	.5/2.3	0	0	0	323	na	0	48
Roast, lean, shoulder	3 oz.	196	11.5/4	.9/5	0	0	0	298	na	0	68
Spareribs, lean	1 med. cut	161	7/3	na	0	0	0	na	na	0	na
Tenderloin, baked	3 oz.	147	5/2	.46/2	0	0	0	368	na	0	47
Bacon, Canadian style	2 slices	86	4/1.3	.45/1.9	0	1.07	0	209	na	0	762
Pork feet, pickled	1 oz.	75	5/2	.48/2	0	.04	0	67	na	0	262
Tongue, braised	3 oz.	230	16/5.5	1.6/7.4	0	0	0	201	na	0	93

Food	Serving Size	Calories	Fat/Sat. Fat (gm)	Poly/Mono Fat (gm)	Fiber (gm)	Sugars (gm)	Carotenoids (mcg or mg)	Potassium (mg)	*Omega-3 Fat	Trans Fat	Sodium
PUDDING											
Banana:											
Instant, prep. w/2% milk	½ cup	153	2.5/1.5	.17/.67	0	28.6	na	190	na	0	429
Instant, sugar-free, prep. w/2% milk (Jello)	½ cup	80	2/0	na	0	na	9 mcg (BC)	na	na	0	na
Ready to eat	½ cup	158	6/2	na	0	na	13 mcg (BC)	na	na	+	na
Regular, prep. w/2% milk	½ cup	143	2.4/1.5	.13/.69	0	27.6	na	206	na	0	246
Bread pudding, w/raisins	1 cup	310	10/3.4	na	2	na	49 mcg (BC)	na	na	un	na
Butterscotch:											
Instant, sugar-free, prep. w/2% milk (Jello)	½ cup	90	2/0	na	0	na	9 mcg (BC)	na	na	0	na
Low-calorie, prep. w/skim milk (D-Zerta)	½ cup	70	0/0	na	0	na	na	na	na	0	na
Ready to eat (Musselman's)	½ cup	170	7/0	na	0	na	13 mcg (BC)	na	na	un	na
Ready to eat (Ultra Slim Fast)	½ cup	100	1/0	na	2	na	0	na	na	0	na

200

Food	Serving Size	Calories	Fat/Sat. Fat (gm)	Poly/Mono Fat (gm)	Fiber (gm)	Sugars (gm)	Carotenoids (mcg or mg)	Potassium (mg)	*Omega-3 Fat	Trans Fat	Sodium
Chocolate:											
Instant, prep. w/2% milk	½ cup	150	3/1.6	.2/.37	.6	28.3	na	252	na	0	426
Instant, sugar-free, prep. w/2% milk (Jello)	½ cup	90	3/0	na	0	na	10 mcg (BC)	na	na	0	na
Lower fat (D-Zerta)	1 serving	20	0/0	na	.5	na	0	na	na	0	na
Ready to eat	½ cup	133	4/1	1.4/1.7	1	17.8	13 mcg (BC)	180	na	un	129
Ready to eat, fat-free (Jello)	½ cup	90	.4/.3	na	.8	15.8	0	109	na	0	213
Regular, prep. w/2% milk	½ cup	150	3/2	.1/.8	.5	27.4	na	234	na	0	146
Coconut cream:											
Instant, prep. w/2% milk	½ cup	157	3.4/2	.28/.9	.15	28.2	na	194	na	0	362
Regular, prep. w/2% milk	½ cup	146	3.5/2.5	.1/.7	.3	24.9	na	223	na	0	228
Custard:											
Mix, prep. w/2% milk	½ cup	149	4/2	.06/.47	0	18.8	na	163	na	0	113
Mix, prep. w/whole milk (Royal)	½ cup	150	5/0	.1/.8	0	18.7	12 mcg (BC)	160	na	0	112
Lemon:											
Instant, prep. w/2% milk	½ cup	154	2.5/1.5	.15/.73	0	30.3	na	195	na	0	402

201

Food	Serving Size	Calories	Fat/Sat. Fat (gm)	Poly/Mono Fat (gm)	Fiber (gm)	Sugars (gm)	Carotenoids (mcg or mg)	Potassium (mg)	*Omega-3 Fat	Trans Fat	Sodium
Ready to eat	½ cup	138	3/1	1.1/1.3	0	25	13 mcg (BC)	1	na	+	140
Regular, prep. w/whole milk (Royal)	½ cup	160	3/0	na	0	na	na	na	na	0	na
Medical Puddings:											
Boost Pudding	5 oz.	240	9/1.5	na	0	na	na	na	na	0	na
Ensure Pudding	4 oz.	170	5/1	na	na	na	na	na	na	0	na
Pistachio:											
Instant, prep. w/whole milk (Jello)	½ cup	170	5/0	na	0	na	na	na	na	0	na
Instant, sugar-free, prep. w/2% milk (Jello)	½ cup	90	3/0	na	0	na	9 mcg (BC)	na	na	0	na
Rice:											
Ready to eat	can	231	10/1.6	4/4.5	0	31	11 mcg (BC)	85	na	+	121
Regular, prep. w/2% milk	½ cup	161	2.3/1.5	.09/.6	.15	31	11 mcg (BC)	195	na	0	164
Tapioca:											
Light, ready to eat (Swiss Miss)	½ cup	100	2/0	na	0	na	na	na	na	0	na
Nonfat, ready to eat (Snack Pack)	½ cup	94	.4/0	na	0	na	0	na	na	0	na
Ready to eat, regular (Lucky Leaf)	½ cup	140	6/0	na	0	na	9 mcg (BC)	na	na	+	na

Food	Serving Size	Calories	Fat/Sat. Fat (gm)	Poly/Mono Fat (gm)	Fiber (gm)	Sugars (gm)	Carotenoids (mcg or mg)	Potassium (mg)	*Omega-3 Fat	Trans Fat	Sodium
Regular, prep. w/2% milk	½ cup	147	2.4/1.5	.08/.6	0	27.3	na	186	na	0	169
Vanilla:											
Instant, sugar-free, prep. w/2% milk (Jello)	½ cup	90	2/0	na	0	na	na	na	na	0	na
Low-calorie, prep. w/ nonfat milk (D-Zerta)	½ cup	70	0/0	na	0	na	9 mcg (BC)	na	na	0	na
Ready to eat	snack size (4 oz.)	181	5/.8	.9/2.1	0	30.6	13 mcg (BC)	158	na	+	189
Ready to eat, fat-free (Jello)	½ cup	92	.2/.2	na	.1	na	0	na	na	0	na
Ready to eat, light (Ultra Slim Fast)	½ cup	100	1/0	na	2	na	0	na	na	0	na
Regular, prep. w/2% milk	½ cup	141	2.4/1.5	na	0	na	na	na	na	0	na
**SALADS											
7-layer salad	1 cup	197	14/4	na	2	12.8	169 mcg (BC)	155	na	0	330
Apple salad	1 cup	192	13/2	na	3*SOL	10.4	49 mcg (BC)	104	na	0	77
Bean salad	1 cup	70	4/.6	na	3*SOL	7.4	48 mcg (BC)	123	high	0	260

**All salads are prepared with fat-based dressings, unless otherwise specified.

203

Food	Serving Size	Calories	Fat/Sat. Fat (gm)	Poly/Mono Fat (gm)	Fiber (gm)	Sugars (gm)	Carotenoids (mcg or mg)	Potassium (mg)	*Omega-3 Fat	Trans Fat	Sodium
Broccoli salad w/cauliflower	1 cup	428	37/9	na	3	16.8	293 mcg (BC)	264	na	0	500
Caesar salad	1 cup	168	14/3	na	1.4	6.1	1 mg (BC)	251	na	0	266
Carrot salad w/raisins	1 cup	419	30/5	na	4*SOL	40	16 mg (BC)	599	na	0	248
Chef salad w/o dressing	1 cup	73	4/2	na	.6	na	519 mcg (BC)	na	na	0	na
Chicken salad	5 oz.	290	22/4	na	.5	na	22 mcg (BC)	na	na	un	na
Cobb salad	1 cup	180	15/4	na	2	5.3	595 mcg (BC)	376	na	0	256
Coleslaw	1 cup	271	24/4	na	4	13.5	2.6 mg (BC)	383	na	0	199
Crab salad	5 oz.	211	10/2	na	.5	8.5	24 mcg (BC)	401	high	0	525
Crab salad w/imitation crab	5 oz.	224	9/1	na	.6	21	24 mcg (BC)	322	high	0	560
Cranberry salad, jellied	1 cup	348	12/1	na	5	60.7	55 mcg (BC)	299	na	0	30
Egg salad	½ cup	354	34/6	na	0	1.8	0	110	high	0	281
Fruit salad w/citrus	1 cup	152	8/2	na	3*SOL	21.6	80 mcg (BC);	273	na	0	50
Fruit salad w/o citrus	1 cup	184	8/2	na	4*SOL citrus	30.1	56 mcg (BC)	374	na	0	47
Greek salad	1 cup	106	7/4	na	1	3.3	404 mcg (BC)	181	na	0	410
Ham salad	5 oz.	298	23/4	na	.6	na	26 mcg (BC)	na	na	un	na
Macaroni salad	1 cup	271	9/1	na	2	43	35 mcg (BC)	118	na	un	331
Mixed salad greens, raw, w/o dressing	1 cup	9	.1/0	na	1	1.6	898 mcg (BC)	174	na	0	14

Food	Serving Size	Calories	Fat/Sat. Fat (gm)	Poly/Mono Fat (gm)	Fiber (gm)	Sugars (gm)	Carotenoids (mcg or mg)	Potassium (mg)	*Omega-3 Fat	Trans Fat	Sodium
SALAD DRESSINGS											
Fat-Free											
1000 Island	1 tbsp.	18	.3/0	.1/.55	0	2.7	2.4 mcg (BC)	20	na	0	117
Blue Cheese	1 tbsp.	19	.1/0	.08/.03	.6	3.7	6 mcg (BC)	33	na	0	136
Creamy, various brands	1 tbsp.	12	.6/.4	.25/.11	0	.91	1 mcg (BC)	23	na	0	170
French	1 tbsp.	21	.5/.1	.01/.02	0	2.6	125 mcg (BC)	13	na	0	128
Italian	1 tbsp.	6	.3/0	.03/.03	0	1.2	2 mcg (BC)	14	na	0	158
Mayo-type, various brands	1 tbsp.	12	.4/.1	na	.6	1	0	8	na	0	120
Ranch	1 tbsp.	18	.4/.1	.1/.05	0	.75	0	16	na	0	106
Reduced Calorie											
Blue Cheese	1 tbsp.	15	1.1/.4	.14/.18	0	.58	0	8	na	0	258
Buttermilk	1 tbsp.	31	3/.6	.65/.81	0	.49	1 mcg	20	na	0	140
Caesar	1 tbsp.	16.5	.7/.1	.36/.17	0	2.4	2 mcg	4	na	0	162
Coleslaw, low fat	1 tbsp.	34	3.4/.5	1.3/1.5	0	6.6	0	9	na	0	272
French	1 tbsp.	32	2/.3	1.2/.49	.1	4	127 mcg	13	na	0	160
Imitation Mayonnaise	1 tbsp.	38	3/.4	1.5/.67	0	.63	0	3	na	0	100
Italian	1 tbsp.	28	3/.4	1.6/.65	0	.27	2 mcg	5	na	0	199
Ranch	1 tbsp.	26	2/.2	na	0	.63	0	20	na	0	151
Russian	1 tbsp.	23	.6/.1	.37/.14	.2	3.5	0	25	na	0	139
Regular											
1000 Island	1 tbsp.	59	5.6/.9	2.9/1.3	0	2.4	0	17	na	0	138
Bacon (hot)	1 tbsp.	101	11/1.7	na	0	na	0	16	na	0	163
Bacon & Tomato	1 tbsp.	49	5/.8	2.9/1.3	0	.3	24.6 mcg	na	na	0	na

Food	Serving Size	Calories	Fat/Sat. Fat (gm)	Poly/Mono Fat (gm)	Fiber (gm)	Sugars (gm)	Carotenoids (mcg or mg)	Potassium (mg)	*Omega-3 Fat	Trans Fat	Sodium
Blue Cheese	1 tbsp.	77	8/1.5	4.2/1.8	0	.54	0	6	na	un	164
Boiled, cooked-type	1 tbsp.	25	1.5/.5	.34/.61	0	1.4	118 mcg	19	na	0	117
Caesar	1 tbsp.	78	8.5/1.3	.48/2	0	.19	2 mcg	4	na	0	158
Celery Seed	1 tbsp.	98	9.6/1.2	na	.2	na	58 mcg	na	na	0	na
Coleslaw	1 tbsp.	121	10/1.5	2.9/1.4	0	3.2	3.6 mcg	1	na	0	114
Creamy Italian or Cucumber	1 tbsp.	74	8/1	na	0	na	2 mcg	na	na	0	na
Feta Cheese (Marzetti)	1 tbsp.	80	8.6/1.7	na	0	na	1 mcg	na	na	0	na
French	1 tbsp.	67	6.4/1.5	3.4/1.3	0	2.5	122 mcg	11	na	0	134
Green Goddess	1 tbsp.	78	7.6/1	4.3/1.7	0	1.1	9 mcg	9	na	0	162
Honey Mustard	1 tbsp.	51	3/.3	na	0	na	0	7	na	0	na
Italian	1 tbsp.	69	7/1	1.9/.92	0	1.2	0	7	na	0	243
Mayo-type (Miracle Whip)	1 tbsp.	57	5/.7	2.6/1.3	0	.94	0	1	na	0	105
Mayo-type, cholesterol-free (Miracle Whip)	1 tbsp.	103	12/1.6	na	0	na	0	na	na	0	na
Peppercorn	1 tbsp.	76	8/1.4	4.4/2	0	.33	2 mcg	24	na	0	143
Poppy Seed	1 tbsp.	65	6/.9	na	0	na	0	na	na	0	na
Ranch	1 tbsp.	74	8/1	4.2/1.7	.45	.37	0	9	na	0	122
Russian	1 tbsp.	76	8/1	4.4/1.8	0	1.6	0	24	na	0	130
Sesame Seed	1 tbsp.	78	8/1	3.8/1.8	.1	1.2	3.6 mcg	24	high	0	150
Vinaigrette	1 tbsp.	69	7/1	3.9/2.4	0	.4	0	1	na	0	0

Food	Serving Size	Calories	Fat/Sat. Fat (gm)	Poly/Mono Fat (gm)	Fiber (gm)	Sugars (gm)	Carotenoids (mcg or mg)	Potassium (mg)	*Omega-3 Fat	Trans Fat	Sodium
Yogurt	1 tbsp.	11	.6/.3	na	0	na	2.4 mcg	na	na	0	na
Zesty Italian (Kraft)	1 tbsp.	54	6.5/.5	na	.08	.67	0	4	na	0	253
SANDWICH MEATS, LEAN											
Beef lunch meat, lean	1 oz.	40	2/0	.1/.93	0	0	0	129	na	0	424
Beef, ultrathin roast (Hillshire Farm)	2 oz.	60	3/1	na	0	na	0	na	na	0	458
Bologna, chicken, lean (Ballard's Farm(	1 slice	120	11/4	na	0	1	0	na	na	0	410
Bologna, fat-free (Oscar Mayer)	1 slice	22	.2/t	.04/.06	0	.62	0	44	na	0	274
Bologna, light (Oscar Mayer)	1 slice	60	4/1.5	.46/2.2	0	.78	0	49	na	0	335
Bologna, low fat (Healthy Choice)	1 slice	30	1/.5	na	0	na	0	na	na	0	na
Bologna, turkey	1 slice	56	4/1.5	1/1.8	0	.78	0	36	na	0	338
Chicken breast, roasted (Field Oven)	1 slice	25	0/0	na	0	na	0	na	na	0	240
Chicken breast, honey (Louis Rich)	1 slice	22.5	.25	na	0	na	0	na	na	0	na
Chicken breast, roasted, fat-free (Oscar Mayer)	1 slice	11	.08/.02	t/.02	0	.12	0	41	na	0	161

Food	Serving Size	Calories	Fat/Sat. Fat (gm)	Poly/Mono Fat (gm)	Fiber (gm)	Sugars (gm)	Carotenoids (mcg or mg)	Potassium (mg)	*Omega-3 Fat	Trans Fat	Sodium
Chicken breast, smoked, 97% fat-free (Louis Rich)	1 slice	30	1/0	na	0	na	0	na	na	0	na
Ham lunch meat, 98% fat-free (Healthy Choice)	7 slices	85	1.5/.5	na	0	na	0	na	na	0	460
Ham lunch meat, extra lean	1 slice	37	1.4/.5	na	0	na	0	na	na	0	na
Ham lunch meat, low fat (Oscar Mayer)	1 slice	22	.8/.18	.23/.24	0	.21	0	56	na	0	258
Lunch meat, light (Spam)	2 oz.	140	12/4	na	0	na	0	na	na	0	na
Turkey breast (Butterball)	1 slice	30	1/.3	.5/0	0	1	0	na	na	0	250
Turkey breast (Healthy Choice)	4 slices	60	1.5/.5	na	0	1	0	na	na	0	450
Turkey breast (Land O Frost)	6 slices	40	4/1	na	0	2	0	na	na	0	650
Turkey breast, white (Land O Frost)	8 slices	60	2.5/.5	na	0	0	0	na	na	0	600
Turkey breast (Plumrose)	1 slice	25	.5/0	na	0	0	0	na	na	0	340
Turkey breast (Tyson)	5 slices	50	1/0	na	0	1	0	na	na	0	590

Food	Serving Size	Calories	Fat/Sat. Fat (gm)	Poly/Mono Fat (gm)	Fiber (gm)	Sugars (gm)	Carotenoids (mcg or mg)	Potassium (mg)	*Omega-3 Fat	Trans Fat	Sodium
SAUSAGE, LEAN											
Pork, light	1 link	70	5/0	na	0	0	0	na	na	0	na
Smoked sausage, lowfat (Healthy Choice)	2 oz.	70	1.5/.5	na	0	0	0	na	na	0	na
Turkey, brown & serve	1 link	40	2/.6	.51/.7	.1	0	0	41	na	0	123
Turkey, smoked	1 medium slice	56	4/.1	na	0	0	0	na	na	0	na
Turkey, Polish (Mr. Turkey)	1 oz.	59	4/0	na	0	0	0	na	na	0	na
Turkey and pork	1 patty	77	6/2	.8/2.4	0	0	0	84	na	0	220
Turkey, pork, and beef, lowfat	1 medium slice	58	1.4/.5	.19/.59	0	0	0	139	na	0	454
Turkey, pork, and beef, reduced fat	1 medium slice	137	10/3.5	1.3/4	0	0	0	116	na	0	545
Turkey summer sausage (Louis Rich)	1 oz. slice	55	4/1	na	0	0	0	na	na	0	na
SNACKS											
Chips											
Apple chips (Weight Watchers)	1 pouch	50	1/0	na	0*SOL	na	3 mcg (BC)	na	na	0	na
Banana chips	1 oz.	147	9.5/8	.18/.55	2	.02	46 mcg (BC)	152	na	0	2

209

Food	Serving Size	Calories	Fat/Sat. Fat (gm)	Poly/Mono Fat (gm)	Fiber (gm)	Sugars (gm)	Carotenoids (mcg or mg)	Potassium (mg)	*Omega-3 Fat	Trans Fat	Sodium
Brown rice chips	1 oz.	130	5/0	na	0	na	na	na	na	0	na
Carrot chips	1 oz.	150	9/0	na	0*SOL	na	1.7 mg (BC)	na	na	0	na
Potato chips, baked	1oz.	120	1/0	na	0	1.2	0	180	na	0	229
Potato chips, barbecue, baked	1 oz.	110	1.5/0	na	.7	na	0	na	na	0	1
Potato chips, dietetic (Spicer's)	1 oz.	100	4/0	na	9	.06	0	366	na	0	185
Potato chips, less fat	1 oz.	130	6/1	3.1/1.2	1.7	.06	0	na	na	un	na
Potato chips, unsalted	1 oz.	150	9.8/1.5	2.6/5	1.4	15	0	na	na	un	na
Sea vegetable chips (Eden Foods)	1 oz.	130	5/0	na	0	na	na	na	na	0	na
Tortilla chips, low fat	10 chips	44	.5/0	.29/.17	.5	.09	52 mcg (BC)	27	na	0	2
Tortilla chips, nacho, baked	1 oz.	110	1/0	1/4.3	2	17.7	52 mcg (BC)	61	na	0	201
Tortilla chips, nacho, light	1 oz.	126	4/.8	.6/2.5	1.4	na	na	na	na	0	na
Tortilla chips, nacho cheese, light	1 oz.	120	4/0	na	0	20	na	77	na	0	284
Vegetable chips (Eden Foods)	1 oz.	130	4/0	na	0	na	na	na	na	0	na
Crisps, Curls, or Puffs											
Cheese puffs, corn-based, light	1 oz	122	3.4/.6	1.6/1	3	2	na	81	na	0	364

Food	Serving Size	Calories	Fat/Sat. Fat (gm)	Poly/Mono Fat (gm)	Fiber (gm)	Sugars (gm)	Carotenoids (mcg or mg)	Potassium (mg)	*Omega-3 Fat	Trans Fat	Sodium
Cheese puffs, cheese flavor	1 oz	157	9.7/1.8	1.3/5.7	.3	.8	na	47	na	un	298
Fruit Bars and Snacks											
Apple fruit bar, nonfat (Health Valley)	1 bar	70	0/0	na	2	na	na	na	na	0	na
Apple raisin bar (Weight Watchers)	1 bar	70	2/.5	na	2	na	na	na	na	0	na
Fruit roll, enriched (Sunkist)	1 roll	72	.2/0	na	1.6	17.4	na	na	na	0	23
Fruit roll-up (Betty Crocker)	2 rolls	104	1/.3	.03/.48	na	10.8	10 mcg (BC)	na	na	0	89
Fruit snack bar (Earth Grains)	1 bar	240	3/0	na	0	na	na	na	na	0	na
Yogurt-coated raisins	9 pieces	170	7/5	na	1	na	na	na	na	0	na
Grain Cakes											
Rice cakes:											
Apple cinnamon	1	50	0/0	na	0	na	na	na	na	0	na
Brown rice, multigrain	1	35	.3/.05	.13/.1	.3*SOL	7.2	0	26	na	0	0
Brown rice, plain	1	35	.25/.05	.09/.09	.4	7.3	0	26	na	0	29
Brown rice, rye	1	35	.35/.05	.14/.12	.4	7.2	0	28	na	0	10
Brown rice, sesame seed	1	35	.35/.05	.1/.1	.5	7.3	0	26	high	0	20
Corn (Quaker)	1	35	.2/0	.1/.1	.2	7.3	3.6 mcg (BC)	25	na	0	26

211

Food	Serving Size	Calories	Fat/Sat. Fat (gm)	Poly/Mono Fat (gm)	Fiber (gm)	Sugars (gm)	Carotenoids (mcg or mg)	Potassium (mg)	*Omega-3 Fat	Trans Fat	Sodium
Popcorn											
Microwave, low fat and sodium	100 gm	429	9.5/1.4	3.6/1	14.2	.54	na	241	na	0	491
Popped, air	1 cup	31	.34/.05	.09/1.2	.66	0	na	na	na	0	24
Caramel-coated, with peanuts	¾ cup	113	2.2/na	na	1.1	13.5	na	101	na	0	84
Oil-popped	1 cup	55	3/5	1.5/.9	1.1	.06	na	25	na	0	97
Pretzels											
Plain	10 pretzels	229	2/5	.69/.77	1.7	.16	0	83	na	un	972
Soft	1 pretzel	190	1.9/.43	.6/.66	2	.16	0	55	na	0	870
Whole wheat	2 oz.	206	1.5/.3	.47/.59	0	46.3	na	245	na	0	116
Snack Mixes											
Fruit and nut (Planter's)	1 oz.	150	10/3	na	t	na	na	na	na	+	na
Party mix, lowfat	1 oz.	120	1.5/.0	na	1	na	na	na	na	un	na
Snack mix	½ cup	150	7/1	na	1	na	22 mcg (BC)	na	na	un	na
Snack mix, baked (Ritz)	1 oz.	130	5.2/1	na	0	18	na	78	na	0	356
Snack mix, DOO DADS	1 oz.	130	5/0	na	0	18.5	na	76	na	un	288
Original (Chex Ralston)	¾ cup	120	0/0	na	1	na	na	na	na	0	na
Snack mix, nonfat	½ cup	180	9/1.5	na	2	na	na	na	na	un	na
Snack mix, w/nuts (Pepperidge Farm)	1 oz.	156	7/1	3/2.8	4	.85	5.4 mcg (BC)	93	na	0	117
Snack mix, oriental	½ cup	347	22/4	7.2/9.4	na	na	na	514	high	un	172
Trail mix, regular	½ cup	347	22/6	4.2/7.2	na	33.6	na	514	high	un	8
Trail mix, unsalted	½ cup	285	12/6	3.6/1.7	na	45.9	na	491	high	un	7

SOUPS

Condensed (Prepared with water unless otherwise specified)

Food	Serving Size	Calories	Fat/Sat. Fat (gm)	Poly/Mono Fat (gm)	Fiber (gm)	Sugars (gm)	Carotenoids (mcg or mg)	Potassium (mg)	*Omega-3 Fat	Trans Fat	Sodium
Asparagus, prep. w/milk	1 cup	161	8/3	na	.75	na	285 mcg (BC)	na	na	0	na
Bean w/Pork	1 cup	172	6/1.5	1.8/2.2	9	2.7	532 mcg (BC)	402	high	0	951
Beef Broth	1 cup	60	0/0	0	0	.2	0	37	na	0	1362
Beef & Mushroom, chunky, low sodium	1 cup	173	5.8/4	.17/99	.25	2.1	3 mg (BC)	351	na	0	63
Beef Noodle	1 cup	83	3/1	.49/1.2	.7	1.3	376 mcg (BC)	100	na	0	952
Black Bean	1 cup	116	1.5/.4	.5/.54	4.5	.2	296 mcg (BC)	274	high	0	1198
Broccoli Cheese, prep. w/milk	1 cup	165	10/3.4	3/4	2	1.2	500 mcg (BC)	414	high	0	1366
Celery	1 cup	90	5.6/1.4	2.5/1.3	.7	8.8	180 mcg (BC)	122	na	0	949
Cheese	1 cup	156	10.5/7	.3/3	1	10.5	670 mcg (BC)	153	na	0	958
Chicken Broth	1 cup	38	1.4/.4	.1/.12	0	1.5	0	24	na	0	792
Chicken Gumbo	1 cup	56	1.5/.3	.34/.66	2	2.5	88 mcg (BC)	76	na	0	954
Chicken Mushroom	1 cup	132	9/2.4	2.3/4	.25	9.3	693 mcg (BC)	154	na	0	942
Chicken Noodle	1 cup	75	2.5/65	.55/1	.7	.27	993 mcg (BC)	55	na	0	1106
Chicken Vegetable	1 cup	75	3/.8	.6/17	.7	1.7	1.5 mg (BC)	154	na	0	945
Chicken w/Dumplings	1 cup	96	5.5/1.3	1.3/2.5	.5	.8	309 mcg (BC)	116	na	0	860
Chicken w/Rice	1 cup	60	2/.5	.41/.91	.7	.24	990 mcg (BC)	101	na	0	815
Chili Beef	1 cup	170	6.6/3.3	.27/2.8	9.5	1.3	900 mcg (BC)	525	na	0	1035
Clam Chowder, Manhattan	1 cup	78	2/.4	1.3/.38	1.5	1	828 mcg (BC)	188	high	0	578

213

Food	Serving Size	Calories	Fat/Sat. Fat (gm)	Poly/Mono Fat (gm)	Fiber (gm)	Sugars (gm)	Carotenoids (mcg or mg)	Potassium (mg)	*Omega-3 Fat	Trans Fat	Sodium
Clam Chowder, New England, prep. w/milk	1 cup	164	6.6/3	1/2.2	1.5	3.9	14 mcg (BC)	300	high	un	992
Minestrone	1 cup	82	2.5/.5	1.1/7	1	11.7	1.4 mg (BC) 3.7 mg (LYC)	93	na	0	891
Mushroom, cream of, prep. w/milk	1 cup	203	13.6/5	4.6/3	.5	7.6	14 mcg (BC)	313	na	0	918
Mushroom Barley	1 cup	73	2.3/.4	.7/1	.7*SOL	11.2	3 mcg (BC)	93	na	0	911
Onion	1 cup	58	2/.26	.65/.75	1	3.6	0	67	na	0	1053
Oyster Stew, prep. w/milk	1 cup	135	8/5	.3/2	0	9.8	67 mcg (BC)	235	high	0	1041
Pea, prep. w/milk	1 cup	239	7/4	.5/2.2	3*SOL	32.3	132 mcg (BC)	376	na	0	970
Pea, Split W/Ham	1 cup	190	4.4/1.7	.6/1.8	2.3*SOL	28	1.3 mg (BC)	400	na	0	1007
Pepperpot	1 cup	104	4.6/2	.36/2	.5	.82	521 mcg (BC)	152	na	0	971
Potato, prep. w/milk	1 cup	149	6.5/4	.57/1.7	.5	17	187 mcg (BC)	322	na	un	1061
Shrimp, prep. w/milk	1 cup	90	5/3	.35/.2	.25	5.8	113 mcg (BC)	248	high	0	1037
Tomato, prep. w/milk	1 cup	161	6/3	1.1	3	12.2	436 mcg (BC) 27 mg (LYC)	449	na	0	744
Tomato Beef	1 cup	139	4.3/1.6	1.6	1.5	2.6	322 mcg (BC)	220	na	0	917
Tomato Bisque, prep. w/milk	1 cup	198	6.6/3	.68/1.7	.5	29.4	436 mcg (BC)	605	na	0	1109
Tomato Rice	1 cup	119	3/.5	1.2/1.9	1.5	9.7	712 mcg (BC)	331	na	0	815
Turkey	1 cup	68	2/.6	1.3/.6	.7	8.6	na	76	na	0	815
Turkey Noodle	1 cup	69	2/.6	.49/.8	.8	8.6	173 mcg (BC)	76	na	0	815

214

Food	Serving Size	Calories	Fat/Sat. Fat (gm)	Poly/Mono Fat (gm)	Fiber (gm)	Sugars (gm)	Carotenoids (mcg or mg)	Potassium (mg)	*Omega-3 Fat	Trans Fat	Sodium
Turkey Vegetable	1 cup	72	3/1	na	.5	na	1.3 mg (BC)	na	na	0	na
Vegetable Beef	1 cup	78	2/.8	.12/.8	.5	.98	1 mg (BC)	173	na	0	791
Vegetable Beef Broth	1 cup	82	2/.4	.8/.5	.5	5.1	913 mcg (LYC)	193	na	0	810
Dry Mix (Prepared with water unless otherwise specified)											
Asparagus	1 cup	58	1.7/.05	na	na	na	271 mcg (BC)	na	na	0	na
Bean W/Bacon	1 cup	106	2/1	.16/.93	9*SOL	.6	532 mcg (BC)	326	na	0	928
Beef Noodle	1 cup	40	.8/.25	.17/.35	.75	6	376 mcg (BC)	80	na	0	1042
Beefy Mushroom (Lipton)	1 serving	33	.4/.05	na	.11	1.6	0	na	na	0	645
Beefy Onion (Lipton)	1 serving	25	.6/.14	na	.35	.53	na	na	na	0	607
Broccoli & Cheese (Lipton Cup-a-Soup)	1 serving	67	3/.8	na	.7	2.1	na	0	high	0	545
Cauliflower	1 cup	69	1.7/.25	.64/.74	na	10.7	109 mcg (BC)	105	Na	0	842
Celery, cream of	1 cup	63.5	1.6/.25	.6/.71	na	9.7	180 mcg (BC)	109	na	0	838
Chicken	1 cup	106	5/3	na	.5	na	434 mcg (BC)	na	na	0	na
Chicken Broth, fat-free (Lipton Cup-a-Soup)	1 serving	18	.13/.02	na	t	.23	0	na	na	0	442
Chicken Noodle		55	1.3/.3	.4/.5	.24	1.2	2 mcg (BC)	31	na	0	550
Chicken Pasta, fat-free (Lipton Cup-a-Soup)	1 serving	44	.3/.5	na	.15	na	na	na	na	0	na
Chicken Rice	1 cup	58	1.4/.3	.4/.6	.7	.48	716 mcg (BC)	10	na	0	931
Chicken Supreme (Lipton Cup-a-Soup)	1 serving	90	3.75/1.4	na	.65	na	na	na	na	0	na

Food	Serving Size	Calories	Fat/Sat. Fat (gm)	Poly/Mono Fat (gm)	Fiber (gm)	Sugars (gm)	Carotenoids (mcg or mg)	Potassium (mg)	*Omega-3 Fat	Trans Fat	Sodium
Chicken Vegetable	1 cup	50	.8/.17	.12/3	na	7.8	na	68	na	0	808
Clam Chowder, Manhattan	1 cup	65	1.5/.26	.5/.72	na	10.9	828 mcg (BC)	200	high	0	1343
Clam Chowder, New England	1 cup	95	3.7/.6	na	1	13	0	207	high	un	755
Consomme	1 cup	17	.02/0	0	0	.65	0	57	na	0	3299
Green Pea (Lipton Cup-a-Soup)	1 serving	75	1/.2	na	3*SOL	.88	32 mcg (BC)	na	na	0	520
Herb, Fiesta (Lipton)	1 serving	29	.3/.05	na	.4	.67	na	na	na	0	559
Leek	1 cup	71	2/1	.07/8.6	3	.81	0	89	high	0	965
Lentil (Lipton Homestyle)	1 serving	127	1/.1	na	5*SOL	1.1	1 mg (BC)	na	na	0	753
Minestrone	1 cup	79	2/.8	.1/.74	na	11.9	na	340	na	0	1026
Mushroom (Lipton Cup-a-Soup)	1 serving	60	2/.3	na	.5	1.44	0	na	na	0	608
Mushroom	1 cup	96	5/.8	1.5/2.2	.8	.38	0	200	na	0	1020
Noodle Rings (Lipton Cup-a-Soup)	1 serving	53	1/.4	na	.2	.18	na	na	na	0	557
Onion	1 cup	27	.5/.12	.07/.3	1	1.9	0	64	na	0	849
Onion Mushroom	1 serving	32	.8/.1	na	.32	.06	na	na	na	0	626
Oxtail	1 cup	68	2.5/1	.1/1	.5	2.7	0	83	na	0	1209
Pasta & Bean (Lipton Homestyle)	1 serving	125	1.4/.3	na	4*SOL	na	181 mcg (BC)	na	na	0	na
Pasta, Spirals (Lipton)	1 serving	64	1/.3	na	.4	na	na	na	na	0	na

Food	Serving Size	Calories	Fat/Sat Fat (gm)	Poly/Mono Fat (gm)	Fiber (gm)	Sugars (gm)	Carotenoids (mcg or mg)	Potassium (mg)	*Omega-3 Fat	Trans Fat	Sodium
Pea	1 cup	133	1.6/.4	4.3/.73	3*SOL	1.6	32 mcg (BC)	238	na	0	1220
Potato	1 cup	68	.6/.1	na	1.5	na	0	na	na	0	na
Ramen Noodle (Nissin)	1 serving	190	7/3	.43/2.7	na	27.5	0	na	na	+	487
Savory Herb w/Garlic (Lipton)											
Tomato	1 serving	31	.4/.09	na	.3	.55	na	na	na	0	477
Tomato	1 cup	103	2.4/1	.2/.9	.5	9.9	493 mcg (BC)	294	na	0	943
Tomato Vegetable	1 cup	53	.8/.4	.07/.3	.5	4.1	116 mcg (BC)	104	na	0	1146
Vegetable, cream of	1 cup	105	5.7/1.4	.5/2.5	.7	.44	638 mcg (BC)	96	na	0	1170
Vegetable Beef	1 cup	53	1/.5	.05/.45	.5	.56	1 mg (BC)	76	na	0	1002
Vegetable (Lipton Cup-a-Soup)	1 serving	52	1/.35	na	.3	.4	137 mcg (BC)	na	na	0	518
Vegetable, Spring (Lipton Cup-A-Soup)	1 serving	47	1.2	na	.65	1.2	na	na	na	0	497
Ready-To-Serve											
Bean, home recipe	1 cup	140	.4/.1	na	7*SOL	na	4 mg (BC)	na	na	0	na
Bean, mixed (inc. 15 bean soup)	1 cup	130	1.5/.4	na	6*SOL	na	137 mcg (BC)	na	na	0	na
Bean w/Ham, chunky	1 cup	231	8.5/3.3	na	11*SOL	na	3 mg (BC)	na	na	0	na
Beef Barley, low fat (Progresso Healthy Classics)	1 cup	137	1.7/.7	.22/7	3.6*SOL	17	na	na	na	0	528
Beef Barley (Progresso Healthy Classics)	1 cup	142	2/.75	.25/.69	3*SOL	20	3 mcg (BC)	118	na	0	396
Beef Soup, chunky	1 cup	170	5/2.5	.22/2.1	1.5	1.6	na	336	na	0	866

217

Food	Serving Size	Calories	Fat/Sat. Fat (gm)	Poly/Mono Fat (gm)	Fiber (gm)	Sugars (gm)	Carotenoids (mcg or mg)	Potassium (mg)	*Omega-3 Fat	Trans Fat	Sodium
Beef Stew (Dinty Moore)	1 cup	222	13/6	.66/.5	2.6	2.3	4.2 mg (BC)	na	na	0	984
Beef Stew (Nestle's Chef Mate)	1 cup	191.5	6/2.4	na	3.3	na	na	396	na	0	na
Beef Vegetable, chunky (Campbell's)	1 cup	153	4.4/1.3	1.2/1	na	16	1.5 mg (BC)	na	na	0	868
Beef Vegetable w/Rice, chunky	1 cup	181	5/2.4	na	1.4	na	1.5 mg (BC)	na	na	0	na
Beer Soup, milk-based	1 cup	109	3.6/1.4	na	.6	na	6 mcg (BC)	na	na	0	na
Beet (Borscht)	1 cup	78.5	4/2.3	na	2	na	6 mcg (BC)	na	na	0	na
Broccoli (Progresso Healthy Classics)	1 cup	88	2.8/.7	.57/.9	2.4	13.3	53 mcg (BC)	161	high	0	578
Carrot, milk-based	1 cup	60	1.6/.6	na	1.3*SOL	na	5.3 mg (BC)	na	na	0	na
Carrot and Rice, milk-based	1 cup	88.5	1.5/.6	na	1.3*SOL	na	4.9 mg (BC)	na	na	0	na
Cauliflower, milk-based	1 cup	197	12/4	na	1.5	na	109 mcg (BC)	na	na	0	na
Chicken, chunky	1 cup	170	6/2	na	1.4	na	773 mcg (BC)	na	na	0	na
Chicken Corn Chowder, chunky	1 cup	238	15/4	na	2	na	na	na	na	un	na
Chicken Noodle, chunky	1 cup	393	13/3	3.4/6	3.3	1.2	na	243	na	0	1908

218

Food	Serving Size	Calories	Fat/Sat. Fat (gm)	Poly/Mono Fat (gm)	Fiber (gm)	Sugars (gm)	Carotenoids (mcg or mg)	Potassium (mg)	*Omega-3 Fat	Trans Fat	Sodium
Chicken Noodle (Progresso Healthy Classics)	1 cup	76	1.6/.4	na	1	na	1.4 mg (BC)	na	na	0	na
Chicken Rice, chunky (Campbell's)	1 cup	127	3/1	.67/1.4	1	2	3.5 mg (BC)	108	na	0	888
Chicken Vegetable, chunky, reduced fat and sodium	1 cup	96	1.2/.3	.26/.4	na	15.2	4 mg (BC)	na	na	0	461
Chicken Vegetable w/Potatoes & Cheese, chunky	1 cup	175	12/4.4	na	.8	na	194 mcg (BC)	na	na	0	na
Chicken w/Wild Rice (Progresso)	1 cup	93	2/.6	.5/.98	na	11.9	na	na	na	0	784
Chili Beef	1 cup	192	7/3	na	4.5	na	128 mcg (BC)	na	na	0	na
Chili Con Carne w/Beans	1 cup	255	8/2	1/5.2	8*SOL	28.1	719 mcg (BC)	674	na	0	1043
Chili Con Carne w/o Beans	1 serving	305	20/7.5	.78/8.8	3.7	16	976 mcg (BC)	na	na	0	812
Chili w/Beans (Hormel)	1 cup	240	4.4/1.8	.86/1.7	8.4*SOL	4.6	na	662	na	0	463
Chili w/Beans (Old El Paso)	1 serving	248	10/2	2.2/4.3	10*SOL	21.6	na	na	na	0	588
Chili w/Beans, Vegetarian (Hormel)	1 cup	205	.7/.12	.2/.07	10*SOL	6.2	na	803	na	0	778

Food	Serving Size	Calories	Fat/Sat. Fat (gm)	Poly/Mono Fat (gm)	Fiber (gm)	Sugars (gm)	Carotenoids (mcg or mg)	Potassium (mg)	*Omega-3 Fat	Trans Fat	Sodium
Chili w/o Beans (Hormel)	1 cup	193.5	6.6/2	.85/2.2	3*SOL	3/3	na	349	na	0	970
Chili w/o Beans (Nestle's Chef Mate)	1 cup	430	32/14	1.8/13.6	3	.18	na	530	na	0	1588
Clam Chowder, Manhattan, chunky	1 cup	134	3.4/2	.12/.98	3	19.7	828 mcg (BC)	59	high	0	283
Clam Chowder, New Eng. (Progresso)	1 cup	117	2/5	.42/.67	1	4	5 mcg (BC)	384	high	+	1001
Crab	1 cup	76	1.5/.4	.16/.28	.7	4.2	77 mcg (BC)	346	high	0	506
Cucumber, milk-based	1 cup	197.5	12/4	na	.5	na	155 mcg (BC)	na	na	0	na
Duck	1 cup	410	37/12.5	na	.3	na	t	na	na	0	na
Egg Drop	1 cup	73	4/1	na	0	na	0	na	na	0	na
Escarole	1 cup	28	2/5	37/8	na	1.8	843 mcg (BC)	265	na	0	3864
Fruit Soup	1 cup	176	.2/0	na	4	na	504 mcg (BC)	na	na	0	na
Garbanzo	1 cup	207	3/3	na	9*SOL	na	19 mcg (BC)	na	na	0	na
Garlic Egg	1 cup	180.5	11/2	na	.4	na	0	na	na	0	na
Garlic & Pasta (Progresso)	1 cup	100	1.3/.3	.46/.36	3	2.04	na	299	na	0	450
Gazpacho	1 cup	46	.25/t	t/t	.5	2.2	1.5 mg (BC)	224	na	0	739
Leek, cream of, milk-based	1 cup	172	8/3	na	.5	na	195 mcg (BC)	na	na	0	na
Lentil (Progresso Healthy Classics)	1 cup	126	1.5/.3	.24/.81	6*SOL	20.3	1 mg (BC)	336	na	0	443
Lentil w/Ham	1 cup	139	3/1	.32/1.3	na*SOL	20.2	1 mg (BC)	357	na	0	1319

Food	Serving Size	Calories	Fat/Sat. Fat (gm)	Poly/Mono Fat (gm)	Fiber (gm)	Sugars (gm)	Carotenoids (mcg or mg)	Potassium (mg)	*Omega-3 Fat	Trans Fat	Sodium
Lima Bean	1 cup	111	3/1	na	5*SOL	na	2.5 mg (BC)	na	na	0	na
Macaroni and Potato	1 cup	211	3.3/1.4	na	3	na	23 mcg (BC)	na	na	0	na
Matzo Ball	1 cup	119	5.5/1.3	na	.4	na	0	na	na	0	na
Minestrone (Progresso Healthy Classics)	1 cup	123	2.5/.4	.99/.92	1	20.3	1.2 mg (BC)	306	na	0	470
Minestrone, chunky	1 cup	127	3/1.5	.2/.9	6	4.6	na	612	na	0	864
Onion, cream of, milk-based	1 cup	172	8/3	1.6/1.5	.5	18.3	195 mcg (BC)	310	na	0	1004
Onion, French	1 cup	58	2/3	na	1	na	0	na	na	0	na
Pea, Split (Progresso Healthy Classics)	1 cup	180	2.3/.76	.42/.9	5*SOL	8.8	1.3 mg (BC)	463	na	0	420
Pea, Split w/Ham, chunky	1 cup	185	4/1.6	.58/1.6	4*SOL	4.5	3 mg (BC)	305	na	0	965
Pea, Split w/Ham, chunky, reduced fat	1 cup	185	2.6/.7	.48/.98	na	27	na	na	na	0	833
Pinto Bean	1 cup	191	.7/.1	na	13*SOL	na	0	na	na	0	na
Potato Cheese	1 cup	187	8/4.6	na	1	na	44 mcg (BC)	na	na	0	na
Potato Chowder, chunky	1 cup	192	12.5/4	4.8/5.9	1.5	13.4	46 mcg (BC)	na	na	un	na
Seaweed	1 cup	83	4/1	na	.6	na	125 mcg (BC)	na	high	0	na
Shark Fin	1 cup	99	4/1	na	0	8.2	na	114	high	0	1082
Sirloin Burger Vegetable (Campbell's)	1 cup	185	9/3	.74/1.2	5.5	na	1.5 mg (BC)	na	na	0	na
Spinach	1 cup	204	12/4	na	2	na	3.6 mg (BC)	na	high	0	na

Food	Serving Size	Calories	Fat/Sat. Fat (gm)	Poly/Mono Fat (gm)	Fiber (gm)	Sugars (gm)	Carotenoids (mcg or mg)	Potassium (mg)	*Omega-3 Fat	Trans Fat	Sodium
Sweet and Sour Tomato Garden (Progresso)	1 cup	72	.8/.3	na	1.6	na	187 mcg (BC)	na	na	0	na
Tortilla	1 cup	99	1/.17	.36/1.2	4	5.2	na	304	na	0	480
Turkey, chunky	1 cup	238	14/4	na	1.4	na	106 mcg (BC)	na	na	0	na
Turkey Noodle, chunky	1 cup	134.5	4.4/1	1/1.7	na	na	na	na	na	0	923
Turtle and Vegetable	1 cup	177	5/1.4	na	1.3	14	1.8 mg (BC)	361	na	0	na
Vegetable (Progresso Healthy Classics)	1 cup	118	4/.8	na	.7	na	98 mcg (BC)	na	na	0	na
Vegetable Beef	1 cup	81	1.3/.3	.35/.44	1.5	13.2	1 mg (BC)	290	na	0	466
Vegetable, chunky	1 cup	128.5	2/.65	.33/.65	4.4	9.6	1 mg (BC)	na	na	0	1095
Vegetable, home recipe	1 cup	122	4/.5	1.4/1.6	1	4.4	3.2 mg (BC)	396	na	0	1010
Vichyssoise	1 cup	100	4.5/.9	na	2	na	1.3 mg (BC)	na	na	0	na
White Bean	1 cup	136	5/3	na	.5	na	187 mcg (BC)	na	na	0	na
Wonton	1 cup	242	7/2.3	na	4	na	1.5 mcg (BC)	na	na	0	na
Zucchini, cream of, milk-based	1 cup	182	7/2.3	na	.9	na	511 mcg (BC)	na	na	0	na
	1 cup	169	10/3	na	1	na	203 mcg (BC)	na	na	0	na

SOY FOODS & PRODUCTS

Food	Serving Size	Calories	Fat/Sat. Fat (gm)	Poly/Mono Fat (gm)	Fiber (gm)	Sugars (gm)	Carotenoids (mcg or mg)	Potassium (mg)	*Omega-3 Fat	Trans Fat	Sodium
Natto	2 tsp.	19	1/.1	.56/.22	.5*SOL	.32	0	66	high	0	1
Nuttettes breakfast cereal	½ cup	140	1.5/na	9*SOL	9*SOL	na	na	na	high	0	na
Miso	½ cup	284	8/1.2	4.4/1.7	7*SOL	7.4	74 mcg (BC)	289	high	0	126

Food	Serving Size	Calories	Fat/Sat. Fat (gm)	Poly/Mono Fat (gm)	Fiber (gm)	Sugars (gm)	Carotenoids (mcg or mg)	Potassium (mg)	*Omega-3 Fat	Trans Fat	Sodium
Miso broth	1 cup	85	3.4/.6	na	2*SOL	na	2.7 mg (BC)	na	high	0	na
Soy beans, cooked from dry	1 cup	311	16/2.3	8.7/3.4	11*SOL	5.1	11 mcg (BC)	886	high	0	2
Soy beans, dry roasted, (soy nuts)	½ cup	219	18.6/1.7	9/4	8*SOL	28.1	56 mcg (BC)	1173	high	0	1173
Soy bacon	1 strip	16	1.5/.2	na	.1*SOL	na	3 mcg (BC)	na	high	0	na
Soy buffalo wings (Morningstar Farms)	5 pieces	200	9/1.5	na	3*SOL	na	na	na	high	0	na
Soy Burgers/Patties:											
Generic	1 patty	140	6.3/1	3.7/1	3.2*SOL	na	0	315	high	0	270
Better n Burgers (Morningstar Farms)	1 patty	80	0/0	na	3*SOL	na	na	na	high	0	na
Breakfast Patties (Morningstar Farms)	1 patty	80	3/.5	na	2*SOL	na	na	na	high	0	na
Harvest Burger (Morningstar Farms)	1 patty	140	4/1.5	na	5*SOL	na	na	na	high	0	na
Soybean butter	2 tbsp.	170	11.6/t	na	.3	na	na	na	high	0	na
Soybean butter, roasted	2 tbsp.	170	11/1.5	na	1	na	na	na	high	0	na
Soy cheeses:											
Unspecified	1 oz.	80–110	0–7/t	na	0	na	na	na	high	0	na
Cheddar	1 oz.	40	3/na	na	0	na	na	na	high	0	na
Mozzarella	1 oz.	20	0/0	na	0	na	na	na	high	0	na
Soybean curd cheese	4 oz.	151	9/1.3	5/2	0	na	27 mcg (BC)	224	high	0	23

Food	Serving Size	Calories	Fat/Sat. Fat (gm)	Poly/Mono Fat (gm)	Fiber (gm)	Sugars (gm)	Carotenoids (mcg or mg)	Potassium (mg)	*Omega-3 Fat	Trans Fat	Sodium
Soybean chips w/o salt 1 oz.		152	9.8/1.2	2.6.5	1.4*SOL	na	15	361	high	0	168
Soy cookies (Essensmart):											
Almond Delight	1 ea.	136	4/t	na	1.2	na	na	na	high	0	na
Orange & Raisin	1 ea.	126	2/0	na	1.4	na	na	na	high	0	na
Ginger & Spice	1 ea.	136	4/t	na	1.4	na	na	na	high	0	na
Soy Beverages:											
Genisoy Natural Protein Powder	1 scoop	100	0/0	0	na	na	74 mg	100	high	0	na
Genisoy Shake— chocolate	1 scoop	120	0/0	2	na	na	na	100	high	0	na
Genisoy Shake— vanilla	1 scoop	130	0/0	0	na	na	na	100	high	0	na
Revival Chocolate Daydream, with fructose	1 packet	240	2.5/1	2	na	na	160 mg	na	high	0	na
Chocolate Daydream, unsweetened	1 packet	130	2.5/1	0	na	na	160 mg	na	high	0	na
Slim-Fast Chocolate Delite with soy protein	2 scoops	170	2/1	1	na	na	na	200	high	0	na
Soyamax	2 scoops	106	1.2/na	na	na	na	60 mg	na	high	0	na
Spirutein Shake, cappuccino	2 scoops	100	0/0	0	na	na	16 mg	400	high	0	na

224

Food	Serving Size	Calories	Fat/Sat. Fat (gm)	Poly/Mono Fat (gm)	Fiber (gm)	Sugars (gm)	Carotenoids (mcg or mg)	Potassium (mg)	*Omega-3 Fat	Trans Fat	Sodium
Spirutein Shake, chocolate	2 scoops	99	0/0	5	na	na	15 mg	400	high	0	na
Super-Green Pro-96	2 scoops	100	1/0	na	na	na	12 mcg (BC) 27 mg	na	high	0	na
Ultra Slim Fast with soy protein	1 can	220	1/0	na	2*SOL	1.6	na	200	high	0	na
Soy flour	¼ cup	94	5/6	2.4/.8	4.4*SOL	5	na	528	high	0	3
Soy flour, defatted	⅓ cup	82	.3/t	.13/t	.9	na	na	596	high	0	5
Soy bread	1 slice	69	1/3	na	.9	na	2 mcg (BC)	na	high	0	3
Soy grits, dry	¼ cup	140	6/1	na	6	na	na	na	high	0	na
Soy hot dog	2 ea.	289	1.5–7/1.1	2.3/.3	1.8*SOL	na	0	266	high	0	228
Big Franks (Loma Linda)	1 ea.	110	7/1	na	2	na	na	na	high	0	na
Soy luncheon meat	1 reg. slice	78	4.5/.7	na	1.4	na	0	na	high	0	na
Soy noodles	1 cup	500	.1/0	na	5.5	na	0	na	high	0	na
Soy nuggets	4 large	614	7.2/1.1	4.9/1.2	1.7*SOL	na	0	252	high	0	216
Soy protein, textured	½ cup	80	0/0	0	4*SOL	6.4	na	115	high	0	230
Soy sauce, regular	1 tbsp.	8.5	0/0	0	.1	.3	0	38	high	0	1005
Soy sauce, reduced sodium	1 tbsp.	8.5	0/0	0	.2	na	0	na	high	0	600
Soy sprouts	1 cup	100	6/na	0	2	na	na	32	high	0	na
Soy supplement bars: Black cherry almond (Cliff)	1 bar	250	5/1.5	na	5	20	na	220	high	0	110
Café mocha fudge (Gensoy)	1 bar	230	4/2.5	na	1	18	na	200	high	0	150

Food	Serving Size	Calories	Fat/Sat. Fat (gm)	Poly/Mono Fat (gm)	Fiber (gm)	Sugars (gm)	Carotenoids (mcg or mg)	Potassium (mg)	*Omega-3 Fat	Trans Fat	Sodium
Chocolate Brownie (Cliff)	1 bar	240	4.5/1.5	na	5	20	na	260	high	0	150
Chocolate fudge brownie (Gensoy)	1 bar	240	5/3	na	2	22	na	250	high	0	210
Chunky peanut butter fudge (Gensoy)	1 bar	240	7/2.5	na	2	26	na	270	high	0	130
Cookies and Cream (Gensoy)	1 bar	240	4.5/2.5	na	1	27	na	170	high	0	250
Creamy Peanut Yogurt (Gensoy)	1 bar	250	6/3	na	1	25	na	200	high	0	160
Lemon Poppyseed (Cliff)	1 bar	230	3.5/1.5	na	5	21	na	210	high	0	110
Soy yogurt	1 cup	102–150	2–4/na	na	1*SOL	na	na	na	high	0	na
Tempeh	½ cup	165	9/1.7	1.3/1.9	7*SOL	4.7	na	201	high	0	7
Tempeh burger	1 patty	245	7.4/na	na	.9	na	na	na	high	0	na
Tofu, regular	½ cup	94	6/9	3.3/1.3	1*SOL	2.3	67 mcg (BC)	150	high	0	9
Tofu, firm	½ cup	97–120	6/1	2/1.5	1*SOL	.76	67 mcg (BC)	186	high	0	15
Tofu, silken	½ cup	72	2.4/t	1.5/.5	0	1.27	67 mcg (BC)	194	high	0	36
Tofu, soft	½ cup	86	5/1	2.6/1	0	.87	67 mcg (BC)	149	high	0	10
Tofu yogurt	1 cup	246	4.7/.7	2.7/1	.5*SOL	na	na	123	high	0	92
Tofutti, chocolate	1 cup	359	24/5.2	na	6*SOL	na	11 mcg (BC)	na	high	0	na
Tofutti, flavors, non-chocolate	1 cup	427	30/4	na	1.2*SOL	na	19 mcg (BC)	na	high	0	na

TOMATOES & TOMATO PRODUCTS

Food	Serving Size	Calories	Fat/Sat. Fat (gm)	Poly/Mono Fat (gm)	Fiber (gm)	Sugars (gm)	Carotenoids (mcg or mg)	Potassium (mg)	*Omega-3 Fat	Trans Fat	Sodium
Canned, chopped	½ cup	30	0/0	0	2	7.3	11.25 mg (LYC)	293	na	0	132
Canned, crushed	½ cup	29	.25/0	t/t	1.5	5.6	11.25 mg (LYC)	264	na	0	282
Canned, whole	½ cup	25	0/0	0	1	3	11.5 mg (LYC)	226	na	0	154
Fresh, boiled	½ cup	32	.5/.07	.24/.09	1.3	4.7	360 mcg (BC) 5 mg (LYC)	427	na	0	9
Marinara sauce	½ cup	71	2.6/.4	na	2	na	285 mcg (BC)	na	na	0	na
Marinara sauce (Contadina)	½ cup	80	4/.5	na	2	na	na	na	na	0	na
Marinara sauce (Prego)	½ cup	110	6/1.5	na	3	na	na	na	na	0	na
Paste	½ cup	107	.7/.1	.3/.1	5.4	15.9	1.6 mg (BC)	1328	na	0	1035
Paste, w/o salt	½ cup	107	.6/.13	.2/.08	5.9	13.6	38 mg (LYC)	1328	na	0	128
Pizza sauce (Contadina)	½ cup	34	7/.3	na	1.3	na	512 mg (BC)	na	na	0	na
Puree	½ cup	50	.2/.02	na	2.5	na	21 mg (LYC)	na	na	0	na
Raw, cherry	1 cherry	4	.06/t	.02/t	.2	.45	na	40	na	0	1
Raw, green	1 medium	30	.25/.03	.1/.03	1.4	4.9	na	251	na	0	16
Raw, Italian	1 medium	13	.2/.02	.08/.03	.7	1.6	na	147	na	0	3
Raw, orange	1 medium	18	.2/.03	.08/.03	1	3.5	na	235	na	0	47
Raw, red	1 medium	26	.4/.05	.16/.06	1.4	3.2	483 mcg (BC) 3.7 mg (LYC)	292	na	0	6
Raw, yellow	1 medium	32	.6/.07	.2/.08	1.5	6.3	na	597	na	0	49
Sauce, canned	1 cup	78	.3/.1	.04/.04	1.8	5.2	512 mcg (BC) 22 mg (LYC)	405	na	0	642

Food	Serving Size	Calories	Fat/Sat. Fat (gm)	Poly/Mono Fat (gm)	Fiber (gm)	Sugars (gm)	Carotenoids (mcg or mg)	Potassium (mg)	*Omega-3 Fat	Trans Fat	Sodium
Spaghetti sauce:											
Chunky	½ cup	50	1/0	na	2	na	na	na	na	0	na
Traditional (Ragu)	½ cup	80	2.6/.36	1.3/.54	0	5.4	na	na	na	0	736
Garlic (Healthy Choice)	½ cup	50	1/0	na	0	na	na	na	na	0	na
Homestyle (Hunt's)	½ cup	60	2/3	na	2	na	na	na	na	0	na
Italian (Healthy Choice)	½ cup	40	0/0	na	0	na	na	na	na	0	na
Meat (Contadina)	½ cup	100	3/1	na	0	na	na	na	na	0	na
Meat (Prego)	½ cup	140	6/1.5	na	3	na	na	na	na	0	na
Meat (Ragu)	½ cup	110	5/0	na	0	na	na	na	na	0	na
Meatless	½ cup	48	1/.16	na	na	na	na	na	na	0	na
Mushroom (Healthy Choice)	½ cup	50	.7/0	na	2.3	na	285 mcg (BC)	na	na	0	na
Mushroom (Prego)	½ cup	110	3/1	na	3	na	285 mcg (BC)	na	na	0	na
Mushroom (Ragu)	½ cup	110	2/0	na	0	na	285 mcg (BC)	na	na	0	662
Parmesan w/herbs and cheese	½ cup	72	2/3	1/.4	2	12.4	na	434	na	0	na
Plain	½ cup	140	4.5/1.5	na	2	na	285 mcg (BC) 20 mg (LYC)	na	na	0	601
Ready to serve	½ cup	70	1.6/.19	1.2/.9	.5	11	285 mcg (BC)	470	na	0	13
Ready to serve, no salt	½ cup	45	.24/.03	.03/.8	1.8	5.2	20 mg (LYC)	453	na	0	na
Sausage	½ cup	180	9/2.5	na	3	na	na	na	na	0	na
Tomato and basil	½ cup	110	3/.5	na	3	na	na	na	na	0	na

Food	Serving Size	Calories	Fat/Sat. Fat (gm)	Poly/Mono Fat (gm)	Fiber (gm)	Sugars (gm)	Carotenoids (mcg or mg)	Potassium (mg)	*Omega-3 Fat	Trans Fat	Sodium
Vegetable (Hunt's)	½ cup	62	1/.1	na	2	na	na	na	na	0	na
Vegetable (Healthy Choice)	½ cup	50	.6/0	na	2.5	na	na	na	na	0	230
Stewed	½ cup	35	1.3/2.6	.4/.52	2	na	na	na	125	na	0	na
Sundried	½ cup	70	.8/.1	na	3.3	na	na	na	na	na	0	na
TURKEY											
Roasted:											
Breast (meat/skin)	100 gm	189	7.4/2	1.8/2.4	0	0	0	288	na	0	63
Dark meat	1 cup	262	10/3.4	3/2.3	0	0	0	406	na	0	111
Leg	1 leg	148	7/2	1.9/2	0	0	0	199	na	0	55
Light meat	1 cup	276	12/3	2.8/3.9	0	0	0	399	na	0	88
Giblets:											
Simmered	1 cup	289	17/5.7	1.8/7.2	0	0	0	392	na	0	93
Patty:											
Breaded, fried	1 patty	181	11.5/3	3/4.8	.3	0	0	176	na	0	512
Patty, cooked	1 patty (4 oz.)	193	11/3	na	0	0	0	na	na	0	na
Turkey ham (Louis Rich)	1 deli-thin slice	15	.38/.12	.09/.1	0	.13	0	41	na	0	158
Turkey ham, honey cured (Louis Rich)	1 slice	30	1/0	.3/.5	0	.4	0	80	na	0	312
Turkey ham, smoked (Mr. Turkey)	1 oz.	32	1.3/0	.25/.38	0	.34	0	72	na	0	258

229

Food	Serving Size	Calories	Fat/Sat. Fat (gm)	Poly/Mono Fat (gm)	Fiber (gm)	Sugars (gm)	Carotenoids (mcg or mg)	Potassium (mg)	*Omega-3 Fat	Trans Fat	Sodium
VEAL											
Blade, roasted	3 oz.	158	7/3	.54/2.7	0	0	0	260	na	0	85
Chop, broiled	1 medium chop	232	13/5.6	na	0	0	0	na	na	0	na
Cutlet, broiled	1 cutlet	136	4/1.6	na	0	0	0	na	na	0	na
Cutlet, breaded, fried	1 cutlet	194	8/2.6	na	.3	.57	0	383	na	0	455
Ground, broiled	3 oz.	146	6.4/2.5	.47/2.4	0	0	0	286	na	0	71
Liver, panfried	3 oz.	208	7.2/2.3	1.2/1.3	0	0	0	388	na	0	94
VEGETABLES & LEGUMES **											
Alfalfa sprouts, raw	1 cup	10	.2/.02	na	1	na	na	na	na	0	na
Artichoke:											
Hearts, canned in water	½ cup	44	0/0	0	6	na	na	na	na	0	na
Hearts, cooked from frozen	3 oz.	30	0/0	0	4	.66	na	209	na	0	229
Marinated	½ cup	168	14/2	na	8	na	na	na	na	0	na
Whole artichoke, globe, cooked	1 medium	60	.2/.04	.08/t	6.5	1.19	na	425	na	0	397
Arugula, raw, chopped	1 cup	5	.1/t	.03/t	.3	.2	na	37	high	0	3
Asparagus, cooked:											
Canned spears	6 ea.	21	.7/.2	.3/.02	2	1.14	na	186	na	0	310

*Cooked with salt unless otherwise stated (to reduce sodium, don't use salt when boiling, baking, or frying)

230

Food	Serving Size	Calories	Fat/Sat. Fat (gm)	Poly/Mono Fat (gm)	Fiber (gm)	Sugars (gm)	Carotenoids (mcg or mg)	Potassium (mg)	*Omega-3 Fat	Trans Fat	Sodium
From fresh, cuts and tips	½ cup	22	.3/.06	1/t	1.5	2.5	na	271	na	0	3
From fresh, spears	6 ea.	22	t/t	.08/t	2	1.8	na	194	na	0	2
From frozen, cuts and tips	½ cup	25	.4/.1	na	1.5	na	na	220	na	0	7
From frozen, spears	6 ea.	25	t/t	t	2	3.6	na	220	na	0	7
Bamboo shoots, canned, drained slices	1 cup	15	.3/.06	.1/t	1	1.2	na	52	na	0	5
Beans, cooked:											
Adzuki, boiled	½ cup	147	.1/.04	na	8*SOL	28.5	na	612	na	0	9
Black beans, canned	½ cup	114	.4/.1	.1/.03	7.5*SOL	20	na	378	na	0	461
Black-eyed peas	½ cup	na	na	na	na	na	na	na	na	0	na
Chickpeas (garbanzo), canned	½ cup	135	2/.2	.6/.3	7*SOL	27	na	206	na	0	359
Fava, canned	½ cup	135	.2/.04	.11/.6	5*SOL	15.9	na	310	na	0	580
Great Northern, canned	½ cup	91	.5/.1	.21/.2	7*SOL	27.5	na	460	na	0	5
Kidney, boiled	½ cup	149	.4/.06	.2/.29	7*SOL	2.3	na	303	na	0	379
Kidney, canned	½ cup	113	.4/.05	.24/.03	4.5*SOL	.28	na	357	na	0	211
Lima, boiled	½ cup	104	.25/.05	.13/.02	5*SOL	1.39	na	485	na	0	215
Lima, canned	½ cup	105	.4/.08	na	5*SOL	na	na	na	na	0	na
Lima, cooked from frozen	½ cup	88	.3/.06	.14/t	5*SOL	1.14	na	258	na	0	246

Food	Serving Size	Calories	Fat/Sat. Fat (gm)	Poly/Mono Fat (gm)	Fiber (gm)	Sugars (gm)	Carotenoids (mcg or mg)	Potassium (mg)	*Omega-3 Fat	Trans Fat	Sodium
Mung, boiled	½ cup	85	.3/.1	.13/.05	8*SOL	2	na	269	na	0	240
Navy, boiled	½ cup	106	.5/.1	.3/.09	6*SOL	.34	na	354	na	0	216
Navy, canned	½ cup	129	.5/.1	.24/.05	7*SOL	.37	na	377	na	0	587
Pinto, boiled	½ cup	148	.4/.09	.16/.11	7*SOL	22.4	na	373	na	0	203
Pinto, canned	½ cup	117	1/.2	.35/.2	5.5*SOL	.26	na	292	na	0	353
Snap, green string and French style:											
Canned	½ cup	18	.1/.03	.12/t	2*SOL	3.9	na	106	na	0	425
From fresh	½ cup	22	.1/.04	.03/t	2*SOL	.77	na	115	na	0	3
From frozen	½ cup	18	.1/.03	.06/t	2*SOL	.83	na	85	na	0	6
Snap, yellow:											
Canned	½ cup	18	.1/.03	.03/t	2*SOL	3.06	na	74	na	0	1
From fresh	½ cup	22	.1/.04	.03/t	2*SOL	3.9	na	115	na	0	3
From frozen	½ cup	18	.1/.02	.05/t	2*SOL	4.35	na	85	na	0	165
White, boiled	½ cup	125	.3/.08	.25/.05	5.5*SOL	23	na	414	na	0	213
White, canned	½ cup	153	4/.1	.16/.03	7*SOL	28.7	na	595	na	0	7
Bean sprouts (Mung), raw	1 cup	31	.2/.05	na	2	na	na	na	na	0	na
Bean sprouts (Mung), canned	1 cup	15	.08/.02	na	1	na	na	na	na	0	na
Beets:											
Raw	2 ea.	70	.3/.04	.1/.05	5	11	na	533	na	0	128
Canned, sliced	½ cup	26	.1/.02	.04/.02	1.5	4.7	na	126	na	0	165
Cooked from fresh, sliced	½ cup	37	.15/.02	.05/.03	2	6.8	na	259	na	0	65

Food	Serving Size	Calories	Fat/Sat. Fat (gm)	Poly/Mono Fat (gm)	Fiber (gm)	Sugars (gm)	Carotenoids (mcg or mg)	Potassium (mg)	*Omega-3 Fat	Trans Fat	Sodium
Pickled slices	½ cup	74	.09/.01	.03/.02	3	18.5	na	168	na	0	300
Whole, canned	1 cup	51	.3/.03	.06/.03	3	16	na	391	na	0	352
Whole, cooked from fresh	2 ea.	44	.2/.03	.06/.03	2	7.9	na	305	na	0	77
Beet greens, cooked	½ cup	20	.14/.02	.05/.03	2	3.9	1.8 mg (BC)	654	na	0	343
Breadfruit, cooked	½ cup	145	.3/.1	na	7	na	31 mcg (BC)	na	na	0	na
Broccoli, raw:											
Chopped	1 cup	25	.3/.05	.03/.01	2.6	1.5	685 mcg (BC) 2 mg (LU+Z)	278	high	0	29
Spears	2 ea.	18	.05/t	.03/2	2	1	483 mcg (BC) 1.5 mg (LU+Z)	196	high	0	20
Broccoli, cooked from fresh:											
Chopped	½ cup	22	.3/.04	.13/t	2	1	813 mcg (BC) 1.7 mg (LU+Z)	229	high	0	204
Spears	2 ea.	21	.3/.04	.12/.02	2	1	771 mcg (BC) 1.6 mg (LU+Z)	217	high	0	194
Broccoli, cooked from frozen:											
Chopped	½ cup	25	.1/.01	.05/t	2	1.3	920 mcg (BC) 764 mcg (LU+Z)	217	high	0	239
Spears	½ cup	26	.1/.01	.05/t	3	1.3	920 mcg (BC) 764 mcg (LU+Z)	131	high	0	239
Broccoflower:											
Raw	1 cup	20	.2/0	.12/.02	2	3.7	58 mcg (BC)	231	high	0	19
Cooked	½ cup	14	.1/0	na	1.5	na	37 mcg (BC)	na	high	0	na

233

Food	Serving Size	Calories	Fat/Sat. Fat (gm)	Poly/Mono Fat (gm)	Fiber (gm)	Sugars (gm)	Carotenoids (mcg or mg)	Potassium (mg)	*Omega-3 Fat	Trans Fat	Sodium
Brussel sprouts:											
Cooked from fresh	½ cup	32	.4/.08	.2/.03	2	6.7	363 mcg (BC)	247	high	0	200
Cooked from frozen	½ cup	33	.3/.02	.02/.03	3	6.4	1 mg (LU+Z) na	252	high	0	201
Cabbage, common varieties:											
Raw, shredded or chopped	1 cup	22	.2/.03	.04/t	2	2.5	58 mcg (BC) 276 mcg (LU+Z)	172	na	0	13
Cooked, drained	½ cup	17	.3/.04	.07/.01	2	3.5	68 mcg (BC)	105	na	0	183
Cabbage:											
Bok choy, raw, shredded	1 cup	9	.1/.01	.07/.01	.7	.83	na	176	na	0	46
Bok choy, cooked	½ cup	10	.1/.01	.06/.01	1.5	.7	na	315	na	0	230
Cabbage, red:											
Raw, chpped	1 cup	19	.2/.02	.11/.05	1.4	3.5	na	216	na	0	24
Cooked, drained	½ cup	16	.15/.02	.07/.01	1.5	3.5	na	105	na	0	183
Cabbage, savoy:											
Raw, chopped	1 cup	19	.07/t	.03/t	2	1.6	na	161	na	0	20
Cooked, drained	½ cup	17	.05/t	.03/t	2	3.9	na	133	na	0	189
Capers	1 tbsp.	2	.07/.02	.03/t	.3	.04	7 mcg (BC)	3	na	0	255
Carrots:											
Fresh, grated	1 cup	47	.2/.03	.13/.01	3*SOL	5	5 mcg (AC) 9.7 mg (BC)	352	na	0	76
Fresh, whole	1 medium	26	.1/.02	.08/.01	2*SOL	3.3	2.8 mg (AC) 5.4 mg (BC)	230	na	0	50

Food	Serving Size	Calories	Fat/Sat. Fat (gm)	Poly/Mono Fat (gm)	Fiber (gm)	Sugars (gm)	Carotenoids (mcg or mg)	Potassium (mg)	*Omega-3 Fat	Trans Fat	Sodium
Carrots, sliced:											
Canned	½ cup	28	.2/.03	.08/t	2*SOL	3	4.3 mg (AC) 7 mg (BC)	183	na	0	295
Cooked from fresh, drained	½ cup	35	.1/.02	.07/t	2.5*SOL	2.7	3.2 mg (AC) 6.3 mg (BC)	140	na	0	236
Cooked from frozen, drained	½ cup	26	.08/.01	.23/.03	2.5*SOL	2.9	4 mg (AC) 9 mg (BC)	95	na	0	215
Carrots, baby:											
Raw	4 medium	15	.2/.04	.03/t	.7*SOL	1.9	1.7 mg (AC) 3 mg (BC)	na	na	0	31
Cooked from frozen	½ cup	35	0/0	na	2*SOL	na	na	186	na	0	57
Cauliflower:											
Raw	1 cup	25	.2/.03	.1/.01	2.5	2.4	na	303	na	0	30
Cooked from fresh, drained	½ cup	14	.3/.04	.12/.02	2	.87	na	88	na	0	150
Cooked from frozen, drained	½ cup	17	.2/.03	.09/.01	2.5	.94	na	125	na	0	229
Celery:											
Raw	1 medium stalk	6	.06/.02	.03/.01	.7	.73	60 mcg (BC) 93 mcg (LU+Z)	104	na	0	32
Cooked from fresh	½ cup	13	.1/.03	.03/t	1	.11	158 mcg (BC) 188 mcg (LU+Z)	213	na	0	245

Food	Serving Size	Calories	Fat/Sat. Fat (gm)	Poly/Mono Fat (gm)	Fiber (gm)	Sugars (gm)	Carotenoids (mcg or mg)	Potassium (mg)	*Omega-3 Fat	Trans Fat	Sodium
Celeriac root, cooked	½ cup	21	.15/0	na	.5	4.6	na	134	na	0	230
Chard, Swiss:											
Raw	1 cup	7	.6/.01	.02/.01	.6	.4	1.4 mg (BC)	136	high	0	77
Cooked from fresh	½ cup	17	.07/0	na	2	.96	na	480	high	0	363
Chayote:											
Raw	1 chayote	39	.3/.06	.11/.02	3.5	3.8	0	254	na	0	4
Cooked	½ cup	19	.3/.07	na	2	4	na	138	na	0	190
Collards:											
Cooked from fresh	½ cup	25	.3/.04	.16/.02	2.5	4.7	4 mg (BC) 7.7 mg (LU+Z)	110	high	0	239
Cooked from frozen	½ cup	30	.35/.05	na	2.5	.48	na	213	na	0	243
Corn (White):											
Canned	½ cup	66	.8/.1	.25/.15	1.5	20.8	na	195	na	0	286
Cooked from fresh, cob	1 ear	96	1/.2	.54/.3	2	3.6	na	222	na	0	225
Cooked from frozen, cob	1 ear	68	.4/.1	.22/.1	2	14	0	158	na	0	151
Cream style	½ cup	92	.5/.08	.25/.16	1.5	2.8	na	172	na	0	365
Kernels, cooked from frozen	½ cup	66	.35/.05	.2/.2	2	16	na	121	na	0	201
Corn (yellow):											
Canned	½ cup	83	.5/.08	.3/.18	2	3.6	928 mcg (LU+Z)	210	na	0	193
Cooked from fresh, cob	1 ear	83	1/.15	.5/.3	2	2.8	1.4 mg (LU+Z)	222	na	0	225

Food	Serving Size	Calories	Fat/Sat. Fat (gm)	Poly/Mono Fat (gm)	Fiber (gm)	Sugars (gm)	Carotenoids (mcg or mg)	Potassium (mg)	*Omega-3 Fat	Trans Fat	Sodium
Cooked from frozen, cob	1 ear	68	.4/.1	.22/.1	2	2.3	43 mcg (BC)	158	na	0	151
Cream style	½ cup	92	.5/.08	.17/.1	1.5	2.5	na	191	na	0	201
Kernels, cooked from frozen	½ cup	82	.6/.09	.25/.16	2	4.1	64 mcg (BC)	172	na	0	365
Cucumber slices w/peel	1 cup	14	.1/.02	.03/0	.8	.87	143 mcg (BC)	76	na	0	1
Cucumber slices w/o peel	1 cup	14	.2/.05	t/t	1	1.6	37 mcg (BC)	162	na	0	2
Dandelion greens:											
Raw	1 cup	25	.4/.09	.17/t	2	2.1	4.6 mg (BC)	218	na	0	42
Cooked	½ cup	17	.3/.07	na	1.5	1.4	3.7 mg (BC)	122	na	0	147
Eggplant, boiled	1 cup	28	.2/.04	.04/.02	2.5	3.7	na	122	na	0	237
Eggplant, cubed, raw	1 cup	21	.15/.03	.06/.01	2	1.9	na	189	na	0	1
Endive, fresh, chopped	1 cup	8.5	.1/.02	.02/t	1.5	t	480 mcg (BC)	79	na	0	6
Grape leaves, raw	1 cup	13	.3/.05	.15/.01	1.5	.88	2.3 mg (BC)	38	na	0	1
Jicama, raw	1 cup	49	.1/.03	.06/t	6	2.3	na	195	na	0	5
Kale:											
Raw, chopped	1 cup	34	.5/.06	.23/t	1	na	6 mg (BC) 26 mg (LU+Z)	299	high	0	29
Cooked from fresh	½ cup	19.5	.3/.04	.25/.04	1	.8	4 mg (BC) 10 mg (LU+Z)	296	high	0	337
Cooked from frozen	½ cup	19.5	.3/t	.3/.05	1	.87	2.5 mg (BC)	417	high	0	326

Food	Serving Size	Calories	Fat/Sat. Fat (gm)	Poly/Mono Fat (gm)	Fiber (gm)	Sugars (gm)	Carotenoids (mcg or mg)	Potassium (mg)	*Omega-3 Fat	Trans Fat	Sodium
Kohlrabi:											
Raw	1 cup	36	.1/.01	.06/t	5	3.5	na	473	na	0	27
Cooked	½ cup	24	.09/t	.04/t	1	1.8	na	281	na	0	212
Leeks:											
Raw	1 leek, bulb/ lower leaves	54	.3/.04	.15/t	1.6	3.5	na	160	high	0	18
Cooked	1 leek, bulb/ lower leaves	38	.25/.03	.14/t	1	na	na	108	high	0	305
Lentils:											
Cooked from dry	½ cup	115	.3/.05	.17/.06	8*SOL	1.8	na	365	na	0	236
Sprouted	1 cup	82	.4/.04	.17/.06	3*SOL	na	na	248	na	0	8
Lettuce, raw, chopped:											
Boston/butterhead	1 cup	7	.1/.01	.06/t	.6	.52	na	131	na	0	3
Escarole	1 cup	8	t/t	t/t	1	na	na	na	na	0	na
Iceberg	1 cup	7	.1/.01	.05/t	.8	.97	106 mcg (BC) 194 mcg (LU+Z)	102	na	0	7
Looseleaf	1 cup	10	.2/.02	.03/t	1	.28	na	70	high	0	10
Radicchio	1 cup	9	.1/.02	na	.4	.24	na	na	high	0	na
Romaine	1 cup	8	t/t	t/t	1	.56	712 mcg (BC) 1.5 mg (LU+Z)	116	high	0	4
Mushrooms:											
Raw, common types, sliced	1 cup	18	.2/.03	.09/t	.9	1.3	na	60	na	0	220
Canned, common type	½ cup, pieces	19	.2/.03	.09/t	2	1.7	na	101	na	0	332

238

Food	Serving Size	Calories	Fat/Sat. Fat (gm)	Poly/Mono Fat (gm)	Fiber (gm)	Sugars (gm)	Carotenoids (mcg or mg)	Potassium (mg)	*Omega-3 Fat	Trans Fat	Sodium
Caps, pickled	8 ea.	11	t/t	t/t	1	na	na	na	na	0	na
Cooked from raw	½ cup, pieces	21	.4/.05	.14/t	2	1.7	na	278	na	0	186
Oyster, raw	1 large	55	.8/0	na	4	na	na	na	na	0	na
Portobella, raw	3.5 oz.	26	.2/.03	.08/t	1.5	1.8	na	484	na	0	6
Shitake, cooked	½ cup, pieces	40	.2/.04	.02/.05	1.5	10.3	na	85	na	0	174
Shitake, dried	4 mushrooms	44	.15/.04	.02/.05	2	3.4	na	230	na	0	2
Straw, canned	½ cup	29	.6/.08	.24/.01	2	4.2	0	71	na	0	349
Okra:											
Raw	1 cup	33	.1/.03	.03/.02	3	1.2	28 mcg (AC) 432 mcg (BC)	303	na	0	8
Cooked from fresh, sliced	½ cup	26	.1/.04	.03/.04	2	3.6	136 mcg (BC) 312 mcg (LU+Z)	108	na	0	193
Cooked from frozen, sliced	½ cup	34	.1/t	t/t	3	2.6	na	205	na	0	220
Onions:											
Raw	1 medium	42	.2/.03	.1/.04	2	6.8	na	230	na	0	5
Raw, chopped	½ cup	31	.1/.02	.07/.02	1.5	4.7	na	158	na	0	3
Cooked	½ cup	46	.2/.03	t/t	1.5	.34	na	12	na	0	18
Green, spring, chopped	½ cup, bulb/top	16	t/t	t/t	1	1.2	196 mcg (BC)	138	na	0	8
Flakes, dehydrated	1 tbsp.	17	t/t	t/t	.5	1.8	na	81	na	0	1
Palm hearts, canned	1 cup	41	1/.2	.3/.15	3.5	6.7	na	258	na	0	622

Food	Serving Size	Calories	Fat/Sat. Fat (gm)	Poly/Mono Fat (gm)	Fiber (gm)	Sugars (gm)	Carotenoids (mcg or mg)	Potassium (mg)	*Omega-3 Fat	Trans Fat	Sodium
Parsley, raw:											
Chopped	½ cup	11	.2/.03	.04/.09	1	.26	1 mg (BC)	166	na	0	17
Sprigs	5 sprigs	2	t/t	t/t	.1	0	156 mcg (BC)	3	na	0	0
Parsnips, cooked, sliced	½ cup	63	.2/.04	.04/t	3	15.2	na	286	na	0	192
Peas:											
Green, canned	½ cup	59	.3/.05	.14/.03	3.5*SOL	3.5	272 mcg (BC)	147	na	0	214
Green, cooked from fresh	½ cup	62	.2/.04	.08/.01	4*SOL	4.7	na	217	na	0	191
Green, cooked from frozen	½ cup	62	.2/.04	.1/.02	4*SOL	11.4	256 mcg (BC)	134	na	0	258
Pod peas, edible, cooked	½ cup	33	t/t	t/t	2*SOL	na	na	na	na	0	na
Split peas, cooked from dry	½ cup	115	.4/.05	.16/.08	8*SOL	2.8	na	355	na	0	233
Peppers:											
Banana, raw	1 medium	12	.2/.02	.11/.01	1.5	.9	18 mcg (AC) 85 mcg (BC)	118	na	0	6
Chili, green, canned	½ cup	14	.07/t	.1/.01	1	3.2	na	79	na	0	276
Chili, green, raw	1 medium	18	.09/t	t/t	.7	2.3	na	153	na	0	3
Chili, red, canned	½ cup	14	.07/t	t/t	1	1.2	na	68	na	0	428
Chili, red, raw	1 medium	18	.09/t	.1/t	.7	2.4	na	145	na	0	4

Food	Serving Size	Calories	Fat/Sat. Fat (gm)	Poly/Mono Fat (gm)	Fiber (gm)	Sugars (gm)	Carotenoids (mcg or mg)	Potassium (mg)	*Omega-3 Fat	Trans Fat	Sodium
Jalapeno, sliced, canned	½ cup	14	.5/.05	.04/t	3	.48	na	30	na	0	0
Jalapeno, raw	1 medium	18	.1/0	.35/.04	.7	1.5	1.5 mg (BC)	131	na	0	1136
Peppers, sweet, green:											
Raw	1 medium	32	.2/.03	.07/.01	2	2.9	635 mcg (BC)	208	na	0	4
Cooked, chopped	½ cup	19	.1/.02	.1/.01	.8	6.2	na	153	na	0	219
Peppers, sweet, red:											
Raw	1 medium	32	.2/.03	.19/t	.2	5	70 mcg (AC) 2.8 mg (BC)	251	na	0	2
Cooked, chopped	½ cup	19	.1/.02	.09/t	.8	6.2	42 mcg (AC) 1.5 mg (BC)	153	na	0	219
Marinated	1 oz.	10	0/0	0	t	2.7	na	102	na	0	958
Peppers, sweet, yellow:											
Raw	1 large	50	.4/.06	na	2	11.7	223 mcg (BC)	394	na	0	4
Strips	10 strips	14	.1/.02	na	.5	3.3	62 mcg (BC)	110	na	0	1
Potatoes:											
Au gratin	1 cup	323	19/12	2.6/6.3	4	27.6	na	970	na	un	1061
Baked w/skin	1 medium	220	t/t	t/t	5	36.6	0	926	na	0	8
Baked w/o skin	1 medium	145	t/t	t/t	2	33.6	0	610	na	0	8
Boiled w/o skin	1 medium	116	t/t	t/t	2	33.4	0	548	na	0	402
Canned	1 cup	108	.4/.1	.16/t	4	24.5	0	412	na	0	394
French fried from frozen	10 fries	100	4/.6	.39/2.4	2	.8	na	209	na	un	15
Hash browns from frozen	½ cup	170	9/4	1/4	2	1.2	na	340	na	un	27

Food	Serving Size	Calories	Fat/Sat. Fat (gm)	Poly/Mono Fat (gm)	Fiber (gm)	Sugars (gm)	Carotenoids (mcg or mg)	Potassium (mg)	*Omega-3 Fat	Trans Fat	Sodium
Mashed w/whole milk	1 cup	162	1.3/.7	.14/.26	4	3.2	0	622	na	0	634
Microwaved w/skin	1 medium	212	t/t	t/t	5	48.7	0	903	na	0	16
Scalloped (Stouffer's)	½ cup	140	6/1	.24/1.5	2	15.6	na	249	na	un	418
Pumpkin, mashed:											
Canned	½ cup	41	.03/.01	.02/.04	3.5	9.9	6 mg (AC) 8.5 mg (BC)	252	high	0	295
Cooked from fresh	½ cup	25	.08/.04	t/.01	1.5	1.2	na	282	high	0	290
Radishes, raw	½ cup	12	.3/.02	.03/.01	1	1.2	na	155	na	0	23
Rutabaga, cooked, mashed	½ cup	47	.3/.04	.11/.03	2	7.2	na	391	na	0	305
Sauerkraut, canned, low sodium	1 cup	27	.2/.05	.09/.02	4	2.5	na	241	na	0	437
Seaweed, kelp, raw	2 tbsp.	4	.06/.03	t/.01	.13	.06	na	9	high	0	23
Shallots, raw	1 tbsp.	7	.01/t	t/t	t	1.7	na	33	na	0	1
Spinach:											
Raw	1 cup	7	.1/.02	.05/t	1	.13	1.7 mg (BC) 3.5 mg (LU+Z)	167	high	0	24
Canned	½ cup	25	.5/.08	.18/.01	2.5	3.4	5 mg (BC)	269	high	0	373
Cooked from fresh	½ cup	20	.25/.03	.1/t	2	3.4	4.7 mg (BC) 6.3 mg (LU+Z)	419	high	0	275
Cooked from frozen	½ cup	27	.2/.03	.2/0	3	4.9	na	287	high	0	306

Food	Serving Size	Calories	Fat/Sat. Fat (gm)	Poly/Mono Fat (gm)	Fiber (gm)	Sugars (gm)	Carotenoids (mcg or mg)	Potassium (mg)	*Omega-3 Fat	Trans Fat	Sodium
Squash, summer:											
Yellow, raw	1 cup	23	.2/.05	.1/.02	2	2.5	102 mcg (BC) 261 mcg (LU+Z)	296	high	0	2
Yellow, cooked	½ cup	14	.07/.1	.12/.02	1.5	2.3	na	173	high	0	213
Zucchini, raw	1 cup	17	.2/.04	.02/t	1.5	1.5	508 mcg (BC) 2.6 mg (LU+Z)	228	high	0	215
Zucchini, cooked	½ cup	14	.04/t	.09/.02	1.2	2.1	na	325	high	0	12
Squash, winter:											
Acorn, mashed, w/o salt	½ cup	41	.1/.03	.04/t	3	10.8	600 mcg (BC)	322	high	0	4
Butternut, mashed, w/o salt	½ cup	47	.08/.01	.04/t	3	10.7	1.3 mg (AC) 5.5 mg (BC)	291	high	0	4
Hubbard, mashed, w/o salt	½ cup	35	.4/.1	.37/.07	3.5	15.2	na	505	high	0	12
Spaghetto, baked or boiled	1 cup	42	.4/.1	.19/.03	2	10	na	181	high	0	394
Sweet potato:											
Baked in skin	1 medium	117	.1/.03	.1/t	3.5	9.6	11 mg (BC)	542	na	0	41
Canned, pieces	1 cup	344	1/.02	.2/.02	6	10	31 mg (BC)	624	na	0	106
Mashed	1 cup	182	.4/.09	.26/0	3.6	18.8	17 mg (BC)	754	na	0	89
Taro shoots, cooked slices	½ cup	10	.05/.01	.02/t	na	2.2	na	241	na	0	167

Food	Serving Size	Calories	Fat/Sat. Fat (gm)	Poly/Mono Fat (gm)	Fiber (gm)	Sugars (gm)	Carotenoids (mcg or mg)	Potassium (mg)	*Omega-3 Fat	Trans Fat	Sodium
Tomatillos:											
Raw, each	1 medium	11	.4/.05	.14/.05	.7	1.3	na	91	na	0	0
Raw, chopped	1 cup	42	1/.2	.5/.2	2.5	5	na	354	na	0	1
Turnips, cooked, mashed	1 cup	48	.2/.02	.1/.01	5	11.3	na	311	na	0	658
Turnip greens:											
Cooked from fresh	½ cup	25	.3/.08	.07/.01	3	.38	3.7 mg (BC) 7 mg (LU+Z)	146	na	0	191
Cooked from frozen	½ cup	25	.4/.08	.06/t	3	.87	na	51	na	0	205
Water chestnuts:											
Canned, slices	½ cup	35	.04/.01	na	2	na	na	na	na	0	na
Canned, whole	4 ea.	14	.02/t	na	.7	na	na	na	na	0	na
Watercress, raw, chopped	1 cup	4	.03/t	.01/t	.5	.07	na	112	na	0	14
VEGETABLES & LEGUMES, MIXED**											
Broccoli, corn, and red pepper	½ cup	60	1/0	na	3	na	na	na	na	0	na
Brussel sprouts, cauliflower, and carrots	½ cup	40	0/0	na	4	na	na	na	na	0	na

*Cooked with salt unless otherwise stated (to reduce sodium, don't use salt when boiling, baking, or frying)

244

Food	Serving Size	Calories	Fat/Sat. Fat (gm)	Poly/Mono Fat (gm)	Fiber (gm)	Sugars (gm)	Carotenoids (mcg or mg)	Potassium (mg)	*Omega-3 Fat	Trans Fat	Sodium
Cauliflower, zucchini, carrots, red pepper	½ cup	30	0/0	na	2	na	na	na	na	0	na
Corn w/peppers (Mexican corn)	½ cup	89	1/2	na	2	na	136 mcg (BC)	na	na	na	0
Green beans and almonds	½ cup	97	7/.7	na	2	na	190 mcg (BC)	na	na	0	na
Green beans and onions	½ cup	23	.1/0	na	2	na	138 mcg (BC)	na	na	0	na
Green beans and potatoes	½ cup	41	.1/0	na	2	na	143 mcg (BC)	na	na	0	na
Green beans and tomatoes	½ cup	25	.2/0	na	2	na	347 mcg (BC)	na	na	0	na
Mixed vegetables, canned	½ cup	43	.2/0	.1/.01	3	7.5	6 mg (BC)	237	na	0	121
Mixed vegetables, from frozen	½ cup	54	.1/0	t/t	4	11.9	2.3 mg (BC)	154	na	0	247
Mixed vegetables, from frozen California blend (Freshlike)	½ cup	30	0/0	na	t	na	na	na	na	0	na
Mixed vegetables, from frozen Italian blend (Freshlike)	½ cup	30	0/0	na	t	na	na	na	na	0	na

245

Food	Serving Size	Calories	Fat/Sat. Fat (gm)	Poly/Mono Fat (gm)	Fiber (gm)	Sugars (gm)	Carotenoids (mcg or mg)	Potassium (mg)	*Omega-3 Fat	Trans Fat	Sodium
Oriental-style mixed vegetables	½ cup	24	.1/0	na	2	na	348 mcg (BC)	na	na	0	na
Peas and carrots, canned	½ cup	50	0/0	0	t	10.8	na	128	na	0	332
Peas and carrots, from frozen	½ cup	38	.3/.06	.16/.03	t	8.1	na	126	na	0	243
Peas and corn	½ cup	78	.6/.1	na	3	na	198 mcg (BC)	na	na	0	na
Peas and mushrooms	½ cup	54	.2/0	na	4	na	258 mcg (BC)	na	na	0	na
Peas and onions	½ cup	41	.2/0	na	2	na	189 mcg (BC)	na	na	0	na
Peas and potatoes	½ cup	67	.1/0	na	3	na	144 mcg (BC)	na	na	0	na
Ratatouille	½ cup	76	6/.8	na	2	na	179 mcg (BC)	na	high	0	na
Succotash	½ cup	89	.9/.2	.4/.15	4*SOL	23.4	132 mcg (BC)	394	high	0	243
Summer squash and onions	½ cup	27	.2/0	na	1	na	102 mcg (BC)	na	high	0	na
Vegetable and pasta combination	½ cup	90	4/1	na	.6	na	1.5 mg (BC)	na	na	0	na
Vegetables, stew type	½ cup	39	.1/0	na	2	na	3 mg (BC)	na	na	0	na
Vegetable stir fry	½ cup	34	.05/0	na	1	na	na	na	na	0	na
Zucchini w/tomato sauce	½ cup	20	.1/0	na	2	na	269 mcg (BC)	na	na	0	na

Food	Serving Size	Calories	Fat/Sat. Fat (gm)	Poly/Mono Fat (gm)	Fiber (gm)	Sugars (gm)	Carotenoids (mcg or mg)	Potassium (mg)	*Omega-3 Fat	Trans Fat	Sodium
YOGURT											
Yogurt, lowfat:											
Fruit flavored	1 cup	250	2.6/1.7	.07/.73	0	46.5	15 mcg (BC)	475	na	0	142
Plain	1 cup	155	3.8/2.5	.1/1	0	17.2	29 mcg (BC)	573	na	0	172
Vanilla, lemon, or coffee	1 cup	209	3/2	.09/.84	0	33.8	15 mcg (BC)	537	na	0	162
Yogurt, nonfat:											
Fruit flavored	1 cup	230	.5/.3	.04/.12	0	46.7	0	478	na	0	142
Fruit flavored (sugar free)	1 cup	122	.4/.2	na	0	17.4	15 mcg (BC)	331	na	0	102
Plain	1 cup	137	.4/.3	.01/.12	0	18.8	0	625	na	0	189
Vanilla, lemon, or coffee	1 cup	223	.4/.3	na	0	na	0	na	na	0	136
Vanilla, lemon, or coffee (sugar free)	1 cup	105	.4/.3	t/.1	0	17.2	0	407	na	0	na
Yogurt, whole milk:											
Fruit flavored	1 cup	291	8/5	na	0	na	47 mcg (BC)	na	na	0	na
Plain	1 cup	150.5	8/5	.22/2.2	0	11.4	44 mcg (BC)	380	na	0	113
Vanilla, lemon, or coffee	1 cup	247	8/5	na	0	na	44 mcg (BC)	na	na	0	na

REFERENCES

Aldana, S.G., *et al.* 2004. The Influence of an Intense Cardiovascular Disease Risk Factor Modification Program. *Prev Cardiol.* 7;1:19–25.

American Diabetes Association. 2004. Reading Food Labels: A Handbook for People with Diabetes. Online: *www.diabetes.org*.

American Heart Association. 1996. AHA Scientific Advisory: Alcohol and Heart Disease, #71-0097 Circulation. 1996;94:3023–3025.

American Heart Association. 2001. AHA Scientific Advisory: Wine and Your Heart, #71-0199 Circulation. 2001;103:472–475.

American Heart Association. 2004. An Eating Plan for Healthy Americans: Our American Heart Association Diet. Online: *www.americanheart.org*.

American Heart Association. 2004. Heart Disease and Stroke Statistics—2004 Update. Online: *www.american heart.org*.

American Heart Association. 2004. Nutrition Facts. Online: *www.americanheart.org.*

American Heart Association. 2004. Nutrition Labeling. Online: *www.americanheart.org.*

American Heart Association. 2004. Dietary Guidelines for Americans. Online: *www.americanheart.org.*

American Heart Association. 2004. Dietary/Lifestyle Interventions and American Heart Association Diets. Online: *www.americanheart.org.*

American Heart Association. 2000. AHA Scientific Statement: AHA Dietary Guidelines: Revision 200, #71-0193 Circulation. 2000;102:2284–2299; Stroke. 2000;31:2751–2766.

Blaco-Colio, Luis Miguel, *et al.* Conundrum of the "French Paradox" *Circulation* (New York). 103 (25):e132, June 26, 2001.

Brouster, J.P. 1999. Wine and Health. *Heart* (May) 81 (5):459–460.

Center for Science in the Public Interest. 2001. Better than Butter? *Nutrition Action Healthletter* (July/August). Online: *www.cspinet.org.*

Center for Science in the Public Interest. 2001. Label Watch: Ingredient Secrets. *Nutrition Action Healthletter* (July/August). Online: *www.cspinet.org.*

Chalfen, Betsy. 1996. Fats: The Good, the Bad, and the Fake. *Sojourner* (March) 21 (7):20.

CTV news staff. 2004. Trans fat in many restaurant, takeout foods. Online: *www.ctv.ca.*

DeNoor, Daniel. 2003. Many "Healthy Foods" full of Unlabeled Trans Fats. February WebMD News

Archive. Online: *www.webmd.com/contnet.article/60/67183.htm.*

Goldberg, Ira J., M.D., *et al.* 2001. Wine and Your Heart: A Science Advisory for Healthcare Professionals from the Nutrition Committee, Council on Epidemiology and Prevention, and Council on Cardiovascular Nursing (New York). 1003 (2):472–475, January 23, 2001.

Greenwood-Robinson, Maggie, Ph.D. *Foods That Combat Heart Disease* New York: Avon Books: 2003.

Henkel, John. Soy: Health Claims for Soy Protein, Questions about Other Components. 2000. *FDA Consumer Magazine* (May/June). Online: *www.fda.gov.fdac/features/2000/300-soy.html.*

Hiroyasu Iso, M.D., *et al.* 2002. Linoleic Acids, Other Fatty Acids, and the Risk of Stroke. *Stroke: Journal of the American Heart Association* (August 1) 33:2086.

Hu, F.B., and Willet, W.C. 2002. Optimal diets for prevention of coronary heart disease. *JAMA* (November 27) 288 (20):2568–78.

Ka He, *et al.* 2004. Folate, Vitamin B6, and B12 Intakes in Relation to Risk of Stroke Among Men. *Stroke* (Jan 2004); 35: 169–174.

Mitchell, Deborah. *The Trans Fat Remedy: The First Consumer Guide to Your Family's Biggest Health Threat.* Signet: 2004.

Ornish, Dean, M.D. *Dr. Dean Ornish's Program for Reversing Heart Disease: The Only System Scientifically Proven to Reverse Heart Disease Without*

Drugs or Surgery. First Ballantine Books: 1991.

Ornish, Dean, M.D. *Everyday Cooking with Dr. Dean Ornish: 150 Easy, Low-Fat High-Flavor Recipes.* HarperCollins: 1996.

Picard, Andre. 2003. Trans fats almost everywhere, tests find. *The Globe and Mail* (December 8).

Plant–fish oil combination better for female heart disease prevention. 2003. *Heart Disease* (February 20).

Pratt, Steven and Matthews, Kathy. *Superfoods RX: Fourteen Foods That Will Change Your Life.* William Morrow: 2004.

Rosenthal, M. Sara, Ph.D. *The Natural Woman's Guide to Living with the Complications of Diabetes.* New Page Books: 2003.

Rosenthal, M. Sara, Ph.D. *The Skinny on Fat.* Toronto: McClelland & Stewart Ltd: 2004.

Rosenthal, M. Sara, Ph.D. *50 Ways Women Can Prevent Heart Disease.* Los Angeles: Lowell House: 2000.

Rosenthal, M. Sara, Ph.D. 2004. Ethical Issues in Food Labeling. Presented at University of Kentucky Department of Behavioral Science.

Stevinson, C., *et al.* Garlic for treating hypercholesterolemia. A meta-analysis of randomized clinical trials. *Ann Intern Med.* 2000;133:420–9.

Truelson, Thomas, M.D. *et al.* 1998. Intake of Beer, Wine and Spirits and Risk of Stroke: The Copenhagen City Heart Study. *Stroke* (December) 29 (12): 2467–72.

Tunstall-Pedoe, Hugh, *et al.* 1994. Myocardial Infarction and Coronary Deaths in the World Health Organization MONICA Project: Registration Procedures, Event Rates, and Case-Fatality Rates in 38 Populations From 21 Countries in Four Continents. *Circulation* (New York). 90 (1): 583–612 (July).

U.S. Department of Agriculture Nutrient Data Laboratory. USDA National Nutrient Database for Standard Reference, Release 17. Beltsville, Maryland.

U.S. Department of Agriculture. 1998. Carotenoid Database for U.S. Foods.

U.S. Department of Agriculture-Iowa State University. 1999. Database for the isoflavone content of foods.

U.S. Department of Health and Human Services, National Heart, Lung, and Blood Institute. 2004. Facts About the Dash Eating Plan. Online: *http://www.nhlbi.nih.gov/*.

U.S. Food and Drug Administration Center for Food Safety and Applied Nutrition. 2003. Guidance on How to Understand and Use the Nutrition Facts Panel on Food Labels (June 2000; Updated July 2003). Online: *www.cfsan.fda.gov/~dms/foodlab.html*.

U.S. Food and Drug Administration. 2000. Health claim notification for potassium-containing foods. Online: *http://vm.cfsan.fda.gov/~dms/hclm-k.html*.

U.S. Food and Drug Administration. 2004. Heart Health Online: Risk Factors for Cardiovascular Disease? Online: *www.fda.gov/hearthealth/riskfactors/riskfactors.html*.

U.S. Food and Drug Administration. 2004. Heart Health Online: What is Cardiovascular Disease? Online: *www.fda.gov/hearthealth/conditions/cvd-conditions.html*.

Weil, Andrew, M.D. 2004. Health: Margarine Vs. Butter. Online: *www.selfgrowth.com/articles/weil.html*.

Weise, Elizabeth. 2004. Latest consumer hook: Trans-fat-free snacks. *USA TODAY* (April 1).

Willet, Walter C. and Meir J. Stampfer. "Rebuilding the Food Pyramid." *Scientific American* (January 2003).

Yusuf, S., *et al.* 2004. Effect of potentially modifiable risk factors associated with myocardial infarction in 52 countries (the INTERHEART study). *The Lancet* (September 11–17 2004); 937.